DECISION MAKING IN NURSING
Tools for change

DECISION MAKING IN NURSING
Tools for change

JUNE T. BAILEY, R.N., Ed.D.

Assistant Dean, School of Nursing;
Director, Creative Leadership
Development Program,
University of California, San Francisco

KAREN E. CLAUS, Ph.D.

Assistant Research Psychologist and Lecturer,
School of Nursing,
Creative Leadership Development Program,
University of California, San Francisco

With 63 illustrations, including 29 drawings by Bee Walters

THE C. V. MOSBY COMPANY
Saint Louis   1975

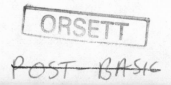

Library of Congress Cataloging in Publication Data

Bailey, June T
  Decision making in nursing.

  Includes index.
    1. Nurses and nursing. 2. Decision making.
I. Claus, Karen E., joint author. II. Title.
[DNLM: 1. Decision making. 2. Nursing, Supervisory.
3. Social change. WY105 B154d]
RT42.B33   610.73   74-28268
ISBN 0-8016-0422-2

GW/VH/VH 9 8 7 6 5

CONTRIBUTORS

EARLINE L. BRYAN, R.N., M.S.
Medical-Surgical Coordinator,
Veterans Administration Hospital,
San Francisco, California

CAROLYN M. FONG, R.N., M.S.
Lecturer, School of Nursing,
University of California,
San Francisco

CARELYN P. FYLLING, R.N., M.S.
Diabetes Nurse Educator and Clinical
Coordinator, Diabetes
Education Center,
Minneapolis, Minnesota

SISTER MARY P. QUAYHAGEN, R.N., M.S.
Lecturer, School of Nursing,
University of California,
Los Angeles

PREFACE

This book is written for all nurses who are concerned with the many dimensions of health care problems and who wish to do something about them. Discrepancies in a health care system that reward illness and discriminate widely have become national issues.

Major beliefs and assumptions about the management of patient care that have influenced our writing and determined the focus of this book are that problem solving and decision making are the central core of management and planned change and that management of health care must move toward a more humanistic adaptive system. We are convinced that change is long overdue. It would seem that nurses who have a history of being advocates for social change and who comprise the largest number of health professionals can be a powerful force in the improvement of the quality and distribution of care. Indeed, nurses can be change agents if they develop their expertise and optimize their power.

The central theme of the book is that to become change agents requires skills and techniques for problem solving and decision making that are basic to management of patient care.

This book is written to provide nurses with practical tools designed to help them solve complex patient-care and management problems and to bring about planned change. This is really a "how to do it" book. We developed a systems model for problem solution over the past 6 years. The primary purpose of the model was one of instruction. It was designed to teach graduate students preparing for leadership roles to become better problem solvers, decision makers, and change agents. The model conceptualizes step-by-step procedures and guidelines for determining overall purposes, goals, and needs of a patient-care or management problem; delineating the problem; analyzing constraints and capabilities; selecting approaches; defining decision criteria; generating alternatives; analyzing options; choosing and implementing a course of action; and evaluating results.

In addition to presenting and discussing the model, the text embodies a series of problems that are presented as case studies. The cases reflect complex problems from the work world that require the nurse to arrive at a solution and to make decisions. Four guest contributors representing a wide variety of practitioner roles in both new and traditional practice settings share their experiences in applying the model to problems in the work locale.

We recognize that processes as complex as problem solving and decision making for nurse managers cannot be learned solely from a book. Knowledge, skills, and understandings acquired by the reader must be put into practice. Our goals are to broaden the perspectives of nursing students and nurse practitioners as to what problem solving and decision making are all about; to present the reader with some analytical tools and techniques that can be applied to improve the quality of patient care through more effective management; and to challenge the reader to test some of the ideas presented here. Hopefully, nurses and other health professionals committed to resolving the health care crisis will begin to play a more creative change-agent role in improving the delivery of health care.

Only when changes are carefully planned to meet the needs of patients, organizations, and health professionals; problems in the health system clearly identified; alternatives creatively generated and analyzed; decisions systematically made; and courses of action implemented and evaluated can the management of patient care move toward a more humanistic, democratic ideal.

The award of a nursing special project grant* to the University of California, San Francisco, made this book possible. We gratefully acknowledge the Public Health Service and the University for the opportunity to work with students in the Leadership Training Program. Through experiences in the teaching program and a growing concern to meet the educational needs of nurses engaged in new and expanded roles, we were inspired and motivated to write this book.

We wish to extend our warmest appreciation to Mrs. Linda Olson and Mrs. Rowena Bishop for their careful, stimulating, and encouraging critique of the manuscript. Their constructive suggestions from the perspective of a nursing educator and a director of nursing service were invaluable. Mrs. Beth Seibert, Miss Wendy Whiteside, Mrs. Nancy Romer, and Miss Janis Morganthaler deserve special thanks for their assistance in the numerous transcriptions and in the typing of the manuscript.

Finally, we wish to express our indebtedness and gratitude to our families for their tolerance, understanding, and sustained support.

June T. Bailey
Karen E. Claus

---

*"Graduate Training of Nurses for Decision Making in Health Care," Training Grant 09D 000394-04-1, United States Department of Health, Education, and Welfare, Public Health Service.

CONTENTS

PART TWO APPLICATION OF CLAUS-BAILEY MODEL TO NURSING CARE PROBLEMS

DECISION MAKING IN NURSING
Tools for change

PART ONE

A FRAMEWORK FOR DECISION MAKING

. . . There are three kinds of people in the world: those who make things happen, those who watch things happen, those who do not know what's happening.

NICHOLAS MURRAY BUTLER

1 PREPARING THE NURSE FOR DECISION MAKING

Nursing and other health professions across the country are confronted with multiple, complex problems. How to "make things happen" to improve the quality of health care services and how to resolve the crisis in the health care delivery system are indeed grave, national concerns. Escalating costs of health care, inequitable distribution and availability of health services, fragmentation of care, lack of teamwork and quality control, "backward incentives"[6], inefficient use of health personnel, and a system in which long-term catastrophic illness is responsible for 50 percent of the personal bankruptcies filed in the nation are some of the charges leveled against the health care industry.

SOCIETY'S CHANGING HEALTH NEEDS

In addition to discrepancies in the health care system, society's health needs are changing. Increased life expectancy has resulted in a need for increased home care and extended care facilities. Skilled nursing care for the elderly who are often afflicted with long-term or chronic illness is long overdue. Complex medical interventions such as heart and kidney transplants require highly trained nursing specialists with new knowledge and skills. Informed consumers are pressing for the facts about their health status, for a more active role in the health care system, and for more consideration of their basic human rights. A number of hospitals have developed materials which they distribute to patients to help them understand their rights as patients.[1]

MEETING THE HEALTH CARE CRISIS

To meet the crisis in the delivery of health services, solutions to problems must come from *within* the organizations since the discrepancies are primarily caused by problems centered around the way health delivery systems are structured. Administrators, physicians, nurses, other health professionals, and consumers of health care must recognize the problems, feel a need to change, and work together in order to "make things happen" in the delivery of more effective health care services.

To improve *nursing care services,* nurses must begin with patient care problems and

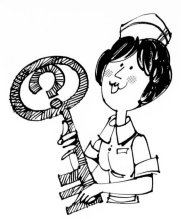

Fig. 1-1. A systematic approach is the key to success in decision making.

needs. A systematic approach is the key to success in decision making. Whenever possible, nurses and patients should solve problems and make decisions together about health care.

An example of developing a system of patient care which started with the needs of patients and which stressed "the human factors in health care" has recently been described by Kraegel and others.[4] This project, carried out by nurses in an acute care center, is indeed a milestone in implementing the concepts of patient-centered care and in using the expertise and scientific knowledge of nurses in the delivery of care.

A number of new models for the organization of health care services have been developed to further meet the needs of patients and consumers of health care. A health maintenance organization model, exemplified by the prepaid group plans of Kaiser Permanente, provides preventive, curative, and rehabilitative care, using ambulatory care facilities. Programs for drug abuse, child abuse, alcoholism, suicide prevention, family planning, and other preventive and health maintenance programs indicate that nursing is assuming a vital role in improving the quality and quantity of health care services and in meeting the changing needs of society.

ACHIEVEMENTS IN NURSING

Major achievements of nurses are further evidenced by the following changes, which are gradually being implemented.

1. *Nursing educational systems* are increasing the number of students, recruiting students from all sectors of society, and preparing students in a wide variety of educational settings for various kinds of practice roles. Provisions are being made for career mobility, credit by examination, acceleration, independent study, and choice of areas of concentration. With emphasis on the problem solving approach,[2] students are encouraged to question, to search, to be innovative, and to evaluate nursing care services.

2. *New and expanded roles* of the nurse have been developed during the last decade. Nurse practitioners, clinical nurse specialists, clinical nurse researchers, primary care nurses, and independent nurse practitioners are expanding the scope of nursing practice. These nurses are committed to using their specialized expertise and are trained to be responsive to the nursing needs of patients.

3. *Nurse practice acts* are being updated to bring "legal definitions of practice in line with the current and projected scope of practice."[3] In 1971, New York and Virginia were

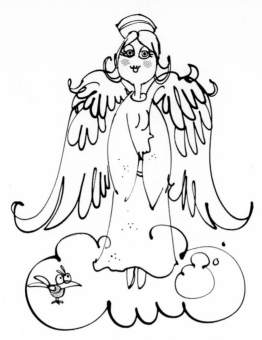

Fig. 1-2. The angel of mercy—new and expanded roles of the nurse have been developed during the last decade.

the first states to update the definition of nursing practice. An ANA survey in 1973 indicated that 30 states have made major amendments or completely revised their practice act during the previous 3 years. Kelly reports that "over the past 10 years, nurses have visibly assumed responsibility for more complex patient care involving major independent decision making. . . ."[3]

4. *Practice settings* are changing. There is a trend toward making health care available in the home and in a variety of community settings other than the hospital. Neighborhood clinics, free clinics, and family clinics exemplify community settings in which nurses are responding to the health care needs of patients.

5. *Health care organizations* are being reorganized. One of the key changes is a "flattening" of the organizational structure and decentralization of authority and decision making. For example, in the vertical structure of hospitals, authority and decision making were highly centralized. With the power for decision making held at the top, it was difficult to retain the patient as a central figure and to achieve the overall purpose of the organization. Changing the structure to a more horizontal format of organization, the power for decision making, responsibility, and accountability is vested in health professionals at the unit level. Primary nursing in acute care centers represents a shift in structure. Although coordinating patient care activities is sometimes more difficult in a horizontal structure, there are many advantages. For example, communication, human relations, and the ability of nursing personnel to function with more autonomy and to use this expertise are decided advantages.

6. *Nursing education systems and nursing service departments* are working more closely together. Recommendations made in the report of the National Commission for the Study of Nursing and Nursing Education have been a primary force in creating more

effective articulation between nursing education systems and nursing service agencies, particularly the hospitals in university health care centers.[7] Joint appointments for nursing educators and nurse practitioners are bridging the gap. A number of medical centers such as Case Western Reserve University and Rush Medical University have developed innovative organizational schemes to relate the educational system to the hospitals' nursing service department.

7. *New modes of organizing nursing care* are exemplified by primary nursing. Marram and others have defined primary nursing as "the distribution of nursing so that the total care of an individual patient is the responsibility of one nurse, not many nurses. Primary nursing can best be differentiated from team or functional nursing, which requires that the total care of any one patient be shared by several nurses during a single shift."[5] A primary nursing system of care is also characterized as a system in which the focus of nursing care is the patient rather than the task.* Since primary nurses are responsible and accountable for making decisions about the nursing care of their patient on a 24-hour basis, nursing is becoming more autonomous and professional.

THE NURSE AS A DECISION MAKER

Inherent in the educational, legal, organizational, and nursing role changes is the expectation that nurses will make intelligent, independent decisions about complex patient care problems and problems related to the delivery of health services. Although many nurses use the nursing process to administer nursing care and are schooled in the scientific method, the growing complexity of problems demands a more rigorous approach. Strategies for nursing action are needed to bridge the gap between problem solving and decision making.

PREPARING THE NURSE TO MAKE EFFECTIVE DECISIONS

The increased decision making responsibilities of the nurse and the expectation that nurses will play a vital role as change agents to improve health services lead to critical questions.

1. Is it reasonable to assume that increasing the clinical expertise of the nurse will also increase the nurse's effectiveness to make intelligent decisions and to be an effective change agent?

2. Can nursing afford to take the consequences if poor decisions are made by nurses who are charged with added responsibility and accountability for decision making?

3. How can nursing be assured that nurses will systematically analyze situations, predict outcomes, make effective decisions, take actions which they can defend, and evaluate the results?

The latter question provided us with the challenge to search for effective ways to conduct seminars on decision making for graduate students enrolled in our Creative Leadership Development Program. A review of the literature on decision theory indicated textbooks and research reports were fraught with complicated mathematical formulas and complex models that proved to be of little value. Frustrations on the part of students and the instructors prompted us to develop a model to assist students in forming a systematic way of thinking about problems and to guide them in the decision making process.

---

*For a more complete discussion of primary care, see Chapter 17.

THE CLAUS-BAILEY MODEL FOR DECISION MAKING*

Experience taught us that a step-by-step procedure conceptualized within a systems framework was an effective way to train nurses to systematically approach problems and to make rational and defensible decisions. In addition, nurses could use their expertise and experience to greater advantage, economize on effort and time, and would be able to more objectively support their decisions.

Although the model contains elements of both systems theory and decision theory, these theories have been adapted and simplified. For example, decision theory does not address itself to problem identification and is concerned primarily with strategies of alternative selection. The model goes back to the beginning and focuses sharply on problem finding and problem definition, areas in which a nurse's expertise is critical. Decision making is viewed as a three-step sequence (search-analyze-choose) and is a central block of activities within the problem solving process.

The model has been tested over a 4-year period. Graduate students have used the model to solve complex problems in various practice settings and have been enthusiastic about the results. (Applications of the model to patient care and nursing service problems are presented in Part two.)

The following chapters discuss in detail the elements and the steps of the model. Each step in the model is presented as a separate chapter. The reader is encouraged to refer to the case studies presented in Part two for detailed examples of how to apply the concepts of the decision making process.

As nurses face the problems inherent in our present health system and search for ways to change it, a systematic procedure embodied in this text may be one way to "make things happen" to alleviate the crisis in the delivery of health care service.

---

*See the inside cover of the book and Chapter 3 for a presentation of the model.

REFERENCES

1. Annas, G. J., and Healey, J.: The patient rights advocate, J. Nurs. Admin. **4:**25-31, 1974.
2. Bailey, J. T., McDonald, F., and Claus, K. E.: An experiment in nursing curriculums at a university, Belmont, Calif., 1972, Wadsworth Publishing Co.
3. Kelly, L. Y.: Nursing practice acts, Am. J. Nurs. **74:**1310-1319, 1974.
4. Kraegel, J. M., Schmidt, V., Shukla, R., and Goldsmith, C. E.: A system of patient care based on patient needs, Nurs. Outlook **20:** 257-264, 1972.
5. Marram, G. D., Schlegel, M. W., and Bevis, E. O.: Primary nursing, St. Louis, 1974, The C. V. Mosby Co.
6. McClure, W.: National health insurance and HMOs, Nurs. Outlook **21:**44-48, 1973.
7. National Commission For The Study of Nursing and Nursing Education: An abstract for action, New York, 1970, McGraw-Hill Book Co.

SUGGESTED READINGS

Abdellah, F. G., Beland, I. L., Martin, A., and Matheney, R. V.: New directions in patient-centered nursing, New York, 1973, The Macmillan Co.

Alexander, E. L.: Nursing administration in the hospital health care system, St. Louis, 1972, The C. V. Mosby Co.

Alexis, M., and Wilson, C. Z.: Organizational decision making, Englewood Cliffs, N. J., 1967, Prentice-Hall, Inc.

Armiger, Sr. B.: Nursing shortage or unemployment, Nurs. Outlook **21:**312-316, 1973.

Arndt, C., and Laeger, E.: Role strain in a diversified role set: The director of nursing service. Part I, Nurs. Res. **19:**253-259, 1970.

Barrett, J.: Administrative factors in development of new nursing practice, J. Nurs. Admin. **1:** 25-29, 1971.

Bennis, W. G., Benne, K. D., and Chin, R., editors: The planning of change, New York, 1969, Holt, Rinehart and Winston.

Board of Directors, National League for Nursing: Nursing education in the seventies, (statement by the Board of Directors, National League for Nursing, approved February, 1972), Nurs. Outlook **20:**271-272, 1972.

Bowman, R. A., and Culpepper, R. C.: Power: Rx for change, Am. J. Nurs. **74:**1054-1056, 1974.

Bridgman, P. W.: Dimensional analysis, New Haven, Conn., 1931, Yale University Press.

Brown, E. L.: Nursing reconsidered: a study of change. Part II: The professional role in institutional nursing, Philadelphia, 1970, J. B. Lippincott Co.

Callow, B.: An R.N.'s view of the health maintenance organization, J. Nurs. Admin. **3:**39-41, 1973.

Chioni, R. M., and Panicucci, C.: Tomorrow's nurse practitioners, Nurs. Outlook **18:**32-35, 1970.

Coombs, C. H.: A theory of data, New York, 1964, John Wiley & Sons, Inc.

Coulter, P. P.: Programming for nursing service, Nurs. Outlook **15:**33-38, 1967.

Donley, Sr. R., Jepson, V., and Perloff, E.: Graduate education for practice realities, Nurs. Outlook **21:**646-649, 1973.

Drucker, P. F.: The effective executive, New York, 1967, Harper & Row, Publishers.

Drucker, P. F.: Management: tasks, responsibilities, practices, New York, 1973, Harper & Row, Publishers.

Dunaye, T. M.: Community planning for new partnerships in health administration, Am. J. Public Health **60:**987-994, 1970.

Easton, A.: Claimantship versus membership as organizational constructs, J. Human Relations **17:**71-76, 1969.

Easton, A.: Complex managerial decisions involving multiple objectives, New York, 1973, John Wiley & Sons, Inc.

Edwards, W. A.: A bibliography of research on behavioral decision processes to 1968, University of Michigan, Human Performance Center, Memorandum Reprint No. 7, 1969.

Elsberry, N.: Power relations in hospital nursing, J. Nurs. Admin. **2:**75-77, 1972.

Ellwood, P. M., Jr.: Concept, organization and strategies of HMOs, J. Nurs. Admin. **3:**29-34, 1973.

Fagin, C. M., and Goodwin, B.: Baccalaureate preparation for primary care, Nurs. Outlook **20:**240-244, 1972.

Forni, P. R.: Trends in licensure and certification, J. Nurs. Admin. **3:**17-23, 1973.

Georgopoulos, B. S.: Hospital organization and administration: Prospects and perspectives, Hosp. Admin. **9:**23-35, 1964.

Good, I. J.: How rational should a manager be? Management Science **8:**383-393, 1966.

Green, B. F.: Current trends in problem solving. In Kleinmuntz, B., editor: Problem solving research, method, and theory, New York, 1966, John Wiley & Sons, Inc.

Hershey, N.: Nursing practice acts and professional delusion, J. Nurs. Admin. **4:**36-39, 1974.

Ingles, T.: Where do nurses fit in the delivery of health care? Arch. Intern. Med. **127:**73-75, 1971.

Jacox, A.: The research component in the nursing service administration master's program, J. Nurs. Admin. **4:**35-39, 1974.

Jones, M. H.: Executive decision making, Homewood, Ill., 1962, Richard D. Irwin Co.

Kirtane, M. V.: Organizational dilemma in hospitals, Hosp. Prog. **55:**49-51, 1974.

Kramer, M.: Team nursing—a means or an end? Nurs. Outlook **19:**648-652, 1971.

Kramer, M.: The consumer's influence on health care, Nurs. Outlook **20:**574-578, 1972.

Kramer, M.: Reality shock—why nurses leave nursing, St. Louis, 1974, The C. V. Mosby Co.

Letourneau, C. U.: New look in hospital organization, Hosp. Management **100:**53-56, 1965.

Lippitt, G. L.: Organizational renewal, New York, 1969, Appleton-Century-Crofts.

Manthey, M.: Primary nursing is alive and well in the hospital, Am. J. Nurs. **73:**83-87, 1973.

Marciniszyn, C.: Decentralization of nursing service, J. Nurs. Admin. **1:**17-24, 1971.

Moral dilemmas for practitioners in a changing society: Editorial (adapted for publication from the Annual Mary Montieth Lecture, April 17, 1972, The Annual Institute of the Loma Linda University School of Nursing Alumni Association, Loma Linda, California), J. Nurs. Admin. **3:**15-17, 1973.

Mulligan, J. E.: There's an HMO in your future: Is your future in the HMO? J. Nurs. Admin. **3:**35-38, 1973.

Mundinger, M. O.: Primary nurse—role evolution, Nurs. Outlook **21:**642-645, 1973.

Munier, S. K., and Richardson, A.: Development of new nursing roles in a comprehensive health center, J. Nurs. Admin. **4:**44-49, 1974.

Nehls, D., Hanson, V., Robertson, P., and Manthey, M.: Planned change: a quest for nursing autonomy, J. Nurs. Admin. **4:**23-27, 1974.

Otto, H. A.: A guide to developing your potential, North Hollywood, Calif., 1973, Wilshire Book Co.

Packer, A. H.: Applying cost-effectiveness concepts to the community health system, Journal of Operations Research Society of America **16:**227-253, 1968.

Pfanzagl, J.: Theory of measurement, New York, 1968, John Wiley & Sons, Inc.

Poulin, M. A.: Nursing service: change or managerial obsolescence, J. Nurs. Admin. **4:**40-43, 1974.

Prest, A. R., and Turvey, R.: Cost-benefit analysis: a survey, Economic Journal **75:**683-735, 1965.

Quinn, N., and Somers, A. R.: The patient's bill of rights: a significant aspect of the consumer revolution, Nurs. Outlook **22:**240-244, 1974.

Robischon, P.: Trends in baccalaureate nursing education, Nurs. Outlook **20:**273-276, 1972.

Rotkovitch, R.: Fifty golden years of education and service: a marriage of convenience or necessity? J. Nurs. Admin. **3:**10-12, 1973.

Schrenk, L. P.: Aiding the decision maker—a decision process model, Ergonomics **12:**543-557, 1969.

Secretary's Committee to Study Extended Roles for Nurses: Extending the scope of nursing practice. Report to the Secretary of Health, Education, and Welfare, Nurs. Outlook **20:**46-52, 1972.

Small, J. E.: Why consider unit management? Hosp. Prog. **55:**74-79, 1974.

Steiner, G. A.: Top management planning, New York, 1969, The Macmillan Co.

Stevens, B. A.: Mandatory continuing education for professional nurse relicensure. What are the issues? J. Nurs. Admin. **3:**25-28, 1973.

Stevens, B. A.: Nursing management and the sense of structure, J. Nurs. Admin. **4:**57-59, 1974.

Stevens, B. A.: The New York state definition of the practice of nursing: implications for nursing education, J. Nurs. Admin. **4:**37-41, 1974.

Tallent, N., Kennedy, G. F., Jr., and Hurley, W. T.: A program for suicidal patients, Am. J. Nurs. **66:**2014-2016, 1966.

Tappan, F. M.: Toward understanding administrators in the medical environment, New York, 1968, The Macmillan Co.

Thomas, L. A.: Action for change: a rationale for nursing administration, Am. J. Nurs. **69:**774-776, 1969.

Valentine, R. F.: Initiative and managerial power, New York, 1973, Amacom.

Williams, K. J.: Beyond responsibility: toward accountability, Hosp. Prog. **53:**44-50, 1972.

Wold, V. C., and Smith, C. M.: Curriculum change: evolution of a dynamic structure, Nurs. Outlook **22:**315-320, 1974.

Zimmern, A., Greenidge, J., and Kohnke, M.: Independent nurse practitioner, Am. J. Nurs. **74:**1093, 1974.

2 APPROACHING PROBLEMS SYSTEMATICALLY

THE IMPORTANCE OF A SYSTEMATIC APPROACH TO SOLVING MANAGEMENT PROBLEMS

All nurses are managers. They may manage the care of a patient or group of patients, a nursing team, a nursing unit, or an entire nursing service. In an educational institution they may manage a school of nursing, a department, or various activities within an educational system. Inherent in the role of the nurse manager* are complex problem solving situations. Although many nurses have been exposed to the scientific method of problem solving, too often problem solving is characterized by unsystematic thinking and unproductive results.

Effective systematic reasoning can be one of the most powerful tools a nurse can use to effect change and to improve the delivery of health or educational services. Indeed, problem solving is the crux of professional practice and decision making is the "hallmark" of a profession.

The nurse's ability to solve patient-centered problems or to assist the patient to solve his own health problems is both immediate and extended by the nature of the situation. Problems may involve providing an educative service such as teaching patients with diabetes how to administer their own insulin. Likewise, nurses are responsible for solving problems that come about as a function of the passing of time, such as those related to the changing nature of patient needs. For example, the needs of patients in an intensive care unit are quite different from the needs of patients when they progress to an extended care facility.

New and extended roles for nurses created to meet patient needs also provide impetus for nurses to become effective problem solvers and decision makers. For example, with the introduction of primary nursing as a mode of nursing care delivery in a number of hospitals across the country, decision making has become decentralized. Primary nurses decide what nursing care their patients need during a 24-hour period and assume the

---

*The terms nurse, nurse manager, and decision maker will be used interchangeably throughout this book.

authority and accountability for making all patient care decisions.[4] In the situations described, the nurse needs to be able to rationally defend the selection of any given course of action. Although the multiple daily work demands of nurses may be such that nurses do not fully use their reasoning processes, systematic reasoning is essential if nurses are to be effective in their extended nursing roles.

The multiple needs of patients, the demands of the health care system for continued nursing services, and the many emergencies that confront nurses require them to act decisively. Nurses who are not versed in the procedures of systematically attacking problems often waste time and energy in making decisions which may be ineffective and

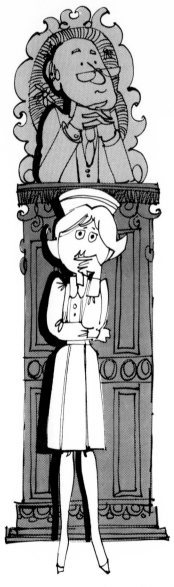

Fig. 2-1. A defensible decision is one that can be explained and whose every step can be recalled if necessary.

which they cannot justify. While this may appear rather academic, nurses are not afforded the luxury of trial and error decision making in patient care settings, even when scant information is available.

The ability to solve problems systematically is equally important to nurses in group situations. In their role as leaders of health care teams, the decision making process of nurses is expanded by virtue of additional input and the dynamics of group interaction. Nurses skilled in making systematic decisions can share their expertise with members of their groups to enhance the ability of group members to make decisions that are defensible.

Defensible decisions

A defensible decision is one that can be explained and whose every step can be recalled if necessary. Whereas once patient care frequently focused on routines and procedures, today's nurse strives to meet the biopsychosocial needs of patients as well as to carry out the technical aspects of care. The nurse is expected to be a problem solver and decision maker in the delivery of patient-centered care.[1] There are many ramifications for this practice, most of which are pragmatic. The application of systematic procedures frees the nurse from distractions that may complicate the task of decision making. Resistance to change on the part of the nursing staff or a nursing faculty exemplifies such a distraction.

Defensible decisions are critical when large expenditures of financial resources are required or when an untoward outcome is irreversible. When the nurse is required to evaluate a procedure or policy, it is also important for her to use a systematic approach so that the rationale can be reconstructed and critically analyzed in open review. The problem of articulating a line of reasoning is simplified through the use of a procedural outline. Such an outline or guide provides nurses with a conceptual framework, which assists them to make sound judgments and to justify their actions.

OBSTACLES TO EFFECTIVE PROBLEM SOLVING

Studies of managerial problem solving indicate that managers often have a tendency to deal with problems, causes, and decisions in a generalized fashion. This procedure may seem necessary when time limitations are imposed; however, if the procedure is adopted and applied to all problem situations, difficulties will be encountered and errors will be made. To illustrate common problem solving difficulties in health care situations, the following examples are presented:

Failing to specify purposes and goals

Evening Supervisor Martha Giles assigned a skilled licensed vocational nurse as head nurse on an intensive care unit of a small 75-bed community hospital for 3 hours when the head nurse went home ill at 8:00 PM. The next day Supervisor Giles was counselled by the Director of Nurses, Mrs. Mary Amy Stevens, for failing to meet the safety and welfare needs of the patients and for failing to comply with hospital policy which required at least one registered nurse on the intensive care unit at all times. Director Stevens pointed out the accreditation of the hospital was in jeopardy and that the registered "float nurse" was employed for the purpose of meeting such emergency situations.

The evening supervisor in the above case failed to specify the overall goals and purposes of nursing care and the purposes of staffing patterns that had been provided. The case demonstrated that the decision the nurse made and the action that was taken to solve the problem were not defensible. In fact, the decision was a poor one, since another

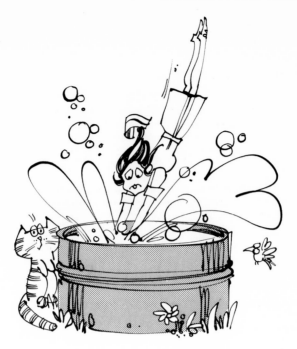

Fig. 2-2. Nurses sometimes plunge into action before considering relevant alternatives.

alternative was available which entailed less risk and which had higher value to patient welfare and safety.

Plunging into action

Assistant Director Alice Martin, a newly appointed supervisor of a 450-bed hospital, was making morning rounds. As she arrived on Station K, Staff Nurse Helen Lyons, was reporting an error she had made in medications to Head Nurse Stacey Davis. Assistant Director Martin hastily announced to those present that in the future any nurse who made an error in administering medications would be fired. Head Nurse Davis, who was on the Hospital Policy Committee, reported the incident to the Director of Nurses, who counselled the Assistant Director and rescinded the order. Ultimately the Assistant Director resigned.

Nurses sometimes plunge into action before considering relevant alternatives. Before making a hasty decision and announcing it, as illustrated in the case which involved an error in administering medications, the Assistant Director should have considered a more effective alternative such as obtaining more information and counselling the nurse in private.

Jumping to conclusions

Director of Nurses Mrs. Jenny Jones denied Staff Nurse Marion Meyers 2 hours of overtime compensation, stating that Nurse Meyers had not obtained permission from the nursing office as required by hospital policy. Nurse Meyers requested an informal grievance hearing. At the hearing, Nursing Director Mrs. Jones discovered that Nurse Meyers had received permission from the head nurse, who was new and stated she did not know that a special form had to be signed by her and submitted to the Director. Nurse Meyers was granted the overtime compensation.

A common error many people make is to jump to conclusions as to the cause of the problem and to proceed on a course of action (often costly) that may or may not solve the problem. The case of denying to pay a nurse for the overtime she worked exemplifies such a misguided course of action.

Failing to look at probable consequences

Nurse Hilda Williams, a staff nurse on the evening shift whose days off were Saturday and Sunday, asked Head Nurse Patricia Parsons on Friday if she could have Monday as an extra day off since her fiance had been granted a three-day pass from the Air Force. Mrs. Parsons granted the request. The following Monday, Head Nurse Parsons realized the unit would be understaffed on the evening shift and that the unit would not meet minimum standards for safe patient care. Mrs. Parsons called a nurse who was on her regular day off and requested that she report for duty since an emergency had arisen. The nurse reported for duty. When she found out that the emergency situation had arisen because of poor planning by the head nurse, she took the incident to the Unit Committee on Grievances.

In the case described, Head Nurse Parsons failed to look at the possible consequences of her actions—inadequate staffing to meet safe patient care standards and a hearing before the Unit Committee on Grievances. The incident illustrated a legitimate complaint of a staff nurse against a head nurse who used the excuse of an emergency situation to cover up a poor management decision.

Errors such as those just described do not necessarily indicate that the nurses were inept. Many errors occur because nurses do not know how to go about systematically gathering information and planning a course of action. Also, nurses often lack clear concepts or a framework from which to approach management tasks.

A conceptual framework provides nurses with step-by-step procedures to guide them in determining what they are tyring to do and how to proceed in an orderly way. Problem analysis and systematic decision making can help accomplish these ends. The nurse at all levels of management needs an orderly and systematic way of progressing through the problem solving process so that decisions are made that can be analyzed and defended.

A SYSTEMS MODEL FOR SOLVING PROBLEMS

One of the major ways in which nurses can make a significant impact in bringing about changes in the health care of society and in the education of nurses is through training them to become better problem solvers and decision makers. Increased knowledge and ability will increase their *expert power* and make them effective change agents.[3] If nurses develop the ability to participate in the problem solving and decision making processes at all levels, things will begin to happen and changes will occur to improve the delivery of health care and the educational instruction of students. A systems model is one way of assisting nurses to become better problem solvers and decision makers.

The nature of a systems approach

Although the term systems is widely used in some disciplines, the systems jargon has had a tendency to turn some nurses off and to create a language barrier between nurses and other management personnel. Concepts of systems theory, however, can be approached and stated rather simply. For example, a system can be conceptualized within a management context as a way of getting something done. A system is a way of thinking and acting which analyzes and integrates knowledge and information for the purpose of improving performance or producing order. All in all, in management, a systems approach usually involves changing or producing something.

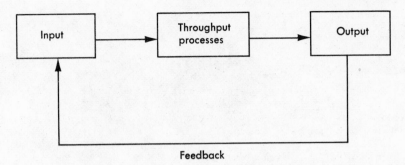

Fig. 2-3. Major elements in a cybernetic model.

Defining a system

A system can be defined as something which is made up of a number of separate parts or elements; the parts or elements of the system rely on each other, are interrelated, have a common purpose, and together form a collective entity or wholeness. Effective systems are characterized by being efficient, reliable, repeatable, and purposeful.

A cybernetic system. The word cybernetic derives from a Greek word meaning helmsman and refers to the guidance or control that a steersman gives to a ship in following a charted course. A navigator (manager) keeps a ship on course by utilizing information about the effects of steering actions (decisions). This knowledge of results is called feedback.[5] A cybernetic system is one which uses feedback to control behavior.

The four major process elements or parts which comprise a cybernetic system are: (1) the inputs; (2) the throughputs or transformation processes; (3) the outputs; and (4) the feedback or knowledge of results. Fig. 2-3 illustrates the relationships among the four process elements.

The importance of feedback. Feedback is information about the consequences of an action which enables a decision maker to correct, supplement, or improve the results of decisions. Feedback provides information about the present state of achievement in relation to the goal. Feedback is also known to serve as a powerful source of motivation to sustain performance and to keep a system operating.[2]

A systems model for the nurse

In developing a systems model for problem solution, we used many of the concepts of systems theory. The model presented in Chapter 3 is a cybernetic systems model with a feedback loop. Nurses who are required to solve problems and to make decisions in the management of patient care need a systems model to help them solve problems and organize tasks, and to provide them with feedback and knowledge of results.

In addition, a cybernetic systems model can provide nurses with an orderly procedure for determining: (1) the goals and expectations of the governing body of a health care delivery system; (2) a clear and precise description of what the current situation is and what it should be; (3) any distinctive discrepancies that can be described; (4) what has changed in the system to cause the problems; (5) possible causes of these problems and the bases for determining probable causes; (6) the decision action that is proposed to remedy the situation; and (7) the means for evaluating the effects of a decision.

ADVANTAGES OF A SYSTEMATIC APPROACH

Expertise in problem solving and decision making gives nurses the following advantages.

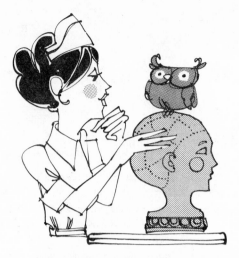

Fig. 2-4. Nurses utilizing a systematic approach have a framework for obtaining relevant information.

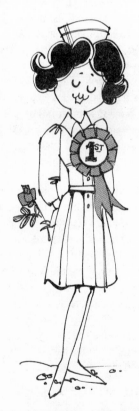

Fig. 2-5. The more systematic the problem solving approach, the greater the opportunity for nurses to utilize their capabilities and potential to the fullest extent.

1. Nurses will know where they are in the problem solving and decision making processes. Step-by-step procedures provide an orderly way to proceed and provide guidelines for analyzing results.
2. Nurses utilizing a systematic approach have a framework for obtaining relevant information. When the process is understood and conceptually clear, nurses will have an orderly way to categorize and use a wide range of relevant information and ideas and will not fall into the trap of gathering data which is irrelevant.
3. A systematic approach to problem solution provides nurses with data for defensible decisions. This is particularly important when large health care expenditures are to be made or when high-risk, high-cost decisions must be made.
4. A systematic approach provides guidelines for making recommendations and bringing about change. When new systems or policies are being considered and nurses at all levels are given responsibility for developing and implementing a major change, this is critical. Furthermore, nurses are expected to instigate and implement change with increasing regularity in institutions across the country. Maintaining the health system as it exists is no longer desirable or defensible.
5. A systematic approach will enable the decision maker to capitalize on experience and resources in order to make better judgments and to defend them. The more systematic the problem solving approach, the greater the opportunity for nurses to utilize their capabilities and potential to the fullest extent.
6. Finally, a systematic approach to problem solving can correct and compensate for errors before the final decision is made and the action taken. Poor decisions, which can be costly, are thus avoided.

The steps outlined in this book will not assure nurses that they will be successful decision makers. No method can guarantee success. The procedures should, however, enable nurses to be more effective and efficient in using the resources at their command, in increasing judgmental skills, in defending the actions that have been taken, and in objectively evaluating the results.

REFERENCES

1. Bailey, J. T., McDonald, F. J., and Claus, K. E.: An experiment in nursing curriculums at a university, Belmont, Calif., 1972, Wadsworth Publishing Co.
2. Bilodeau, E. A., and Bilodeau, I. M.: Motor-skills learning, Ann. Rev. Psychol. **12:**250, 1961.
3. Katz, D., and Kahn, R.: The social psychology of organizations, New York, 1966, John Wiley & Sons, Inc.
4. Marram, G., Schlegel, M., and Bevis, E.: Primary nursing, St. Louis, 1974, The C. V. Mosby Co.
5. Wiener, N.: Cybernetics, New York, 1948, John Wiley & Sons, Inc.

SUGGESTED READINGS

Carlisle, H. M.: Situational management, New York, 1973, American Management Association.
Cloner, A.: The influence of systems theory in educating health services administrators. The University of Southern California experience, Am. J. Public Health **60:**995-1005, 1970.
Emery, F. E., editor: Systems thinking, Baltimore, 1969, Penguin Books.
Gordon, M., and Anello, M.: A systematic approach to curriculum revision, Nurs. Outlook **22:**306-309, 1974.
Hall, A. D.: A methodology for systems engineering, New York, 1962, Van Nostrand-Reinhold Books.
Heimstra, N. W., and Ellingstad, V. S.: Human behavior: a systems approach, Monterey, Calif., 1972, Brooks-Cole Publishing Co.
Mayers, M. G.: A systematic approach to the nursing care plan, New York, 1972, Appleton-Century-Crofts.
Roy, Sr. C.: Adaptation: a conceptual framework for nursing, Nurs. Outlook **18:**42-45, 1970.
Smoyak, S. A.: Toward understanding nursing situations: a transaction paradigm, Nurs. Res. **18:**405-411, 1969.
von Bertalanffy, L.: General systems theory, General Systems, Yearbook of the Society for the Advancement of General Systems Theory **1:**1-10, 1956.

3 A SYSTEMS MODEL TO GUIDE PROBLEM SOLVING AND DECISION MAKING

THE CLAUS-BAILEY PROBLEM SOLVING MODEL

In Chapter 2 a cybernetic system was described as having *input,* which is acted upon or transformed to yield *output.* Critical to the cybernetic system is *feedback,* or information about the results of actions. This feedback serves to guide the system's subsequent actions.

The cybernetic system with a closed feedback loop served as a framework for the development of the Claus-Bailey Model for Problem Solution presented in Fig. 3-1. The model is presented in linear fashion to indicate the various components in the process. The linear steps were developed to present the reader with an overview of the entire process. Such step-by-step procedures enable a decision maker to think systematically. The model provides guidelines so that no steps in the process are omitted, and so that the problem solving situation can be entered at any point in the process.

Nurses are frequently required to enter a problem solving situation somewhere in the middle of the system sequence. For example, nurses sometimes find themselves being added to a task force or to a committee when a problem has already been defined and partially explored by members of the group. The nurse may discover when she joins the group that the members have focused on possible reasons for the problem rather on the problem itself. Previous activities of those concerned with the problem then need to be reexamined. An analytical tool such as presented by the model would enable the nurse and the other group members to systematically retrace activities and to redefine the problem.

THE DYNAMICS OF A PROBLEM

The dynamic nature of the problem solving process is such that any one element may alter the significance of information which has been obtained previously or which will be obtained in the later stages of the process. It is essential to keep this in mind be-

---

*From Drucker, P. F.: The effective executive, New York, 1967, Harper & Row, Publishers, p. 113.

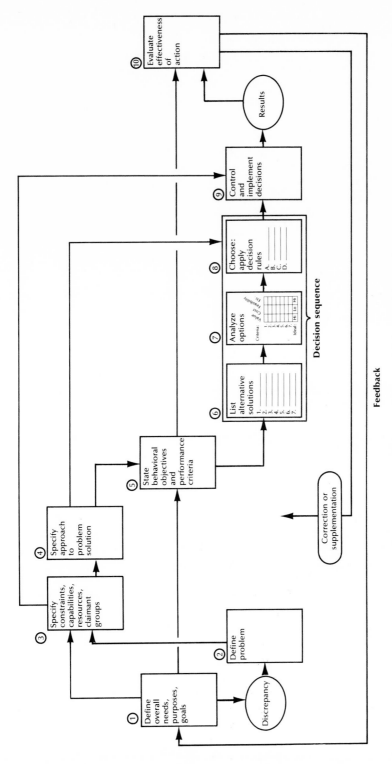

Fig. 3-1. Claus-Bailey systems model for problem solution.

cause the decision maker must be sensitive to element interactions. In effective problem solving certain processes are more directly related to certain other processes. These relationships are indicated by the arrows in Fig. 3-1.

The concepts presented in this chapter are intended to provide the reader with a step-by-step analytical tool and to encourage the reader to use the tool to develop effective systematic reasoning. The order of the ten steps and the relationship between steps are critical factors in understanding and applying the model to a problem solving situation.

In certain problem solving situations such as emergencies nurses must respond quickly. Although experience may provide nurses with insight and assist them in selecting effective nursing interventions, there are pitfalls in making nursing judgments and taking nursing actions based solely on experience. Nurses today are expected not only to make sound judgments, but to account for them. The model presented in Fig. 3-1 provides the nurse with a system for both making judgments and accounting for them.

STEP 1: DEFINE OVERALL NEEDS, PURPOSES, AND GOALS

Define
overall
needs,
purposes,
goals

The first step in the systems model for problem solving is critical to the entire problem solving process. Ideally, definition of overall needs, purposes, and goals should be done before a problem is encountered. However, when a problem is noted, it may be done concurrently. This first step in problem solving is frequently omitted or superficially approached in decision making. Too often only the broadest ideas about goals are stated, such as "To make the patient well," or "To hold down costs." A goal stated in this manner is too vague to be effectively achieved.

Overall purposes and goals are based upon needs. These can be needs of a system, such as a hospital, needs of the individuals within that system, for example, the nurses, or needs of the clients of that system, the patients. In problem solving, the solution is the achievement of a goal. Therefore a goal should encourage generation of precise standards that can be used in analyzing the effectiveness of any given action. When a goal is being formulated, certain questions such as "what kind?" "how much?" "when?" and "where?" should be asked. When goals are stated which follow these guidelines, they can be used as criteria in assessing the quality of the decision making process. Overall needs, purposes, and goals are related directly to the establishment of the problem. If overall needs, purposes, and goals are not spelled out clearly, it is difficult to focus on the exact nature of the problem at hand. Indeed, how can a problem be described and handled when standards are not established?

The nature of a problem—the discrepancy

For our purposes a problem is defined as a *discrepancy*—a discrepancy which exists between what actually is and what should be or could be. The term discrepancy indicates a difference (in this case the difference between what one observes the present situation to be and what one believes is desired). Other terms that may come to mind within this context include deviation, deficiency, and imbalance, but in common usage these terms indicate a value judgment. To avoid emotional overtones suggested by such terms and to avoid drawing conclusions before they are appropriate, we have selected the term discrepancy.

In problems of planning, the discrepancy may be a difference between "what is" and "what should or could be." For example, the discrepancy in an acute care hospital

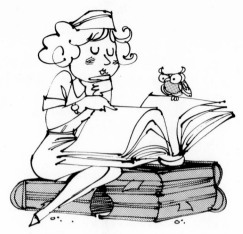

Fig. 3-2. The first step in defining a problem requires that accurate information be collected and used in diagnosing the problem.

may be that there are no quality controls of patient care, although quality controls "should be" an integral part of patient care management.*

STEP 2: DEFINING THE PROBLEM

> Define
> problem

Recognition of a problem implies a desire for change. Someone must generate the pressure for a change in the status quo.

Definition of the problem is the critical second step in the problem solving procedure. The process of problem definition helps decision makers to focus on the correct problem and to conserve time and energy.

The first step in defining a problem requires that accurate information be collected and used in diagnosing the problem. (A clear statement of what "should be" is necessary.) The nurse must collect information that will identify and enumerate the symptoms and clues which could account for the difference. The nurse must then begin to pinpoint the exact nature of the discrepancy. This involves asking very basic questions such as: What is the nature of the discrepancy? What is happening? Where is it happening? Is this situation stable or variable? It is important at this stage to specify the times and places of the symptoms and their occurrence. Recent changes in the system's structure, processes, or environment should be noted and a list of tentative hypotheses regarding the nature of the cause of the discrepancy should be developed. The hypotheses can be tested against the facts which are listed and diagrammed. (This procedure is described in Chapter 5.) Progressive elimination of hypotheses that fail to conform to the facts will eventually yield a hypothesis that does describe the nature of the discrepancy. When a hypothesis is accepted, the nurse should use all available information to determine the validity of the hypothetical cause.

---

*A "should be" statement implies a value judgment that rests upon certain assumptions about what is "good," "appropriate," or "desirable" in terms of functioning. We need to look at the assumptions and values by which we judge behavior or situations; whose values are operating—ours, the client's, the chief financial officer's, and why. This is discussed in Chapter 7.

STEP 3: WEIGHING THE CONSTRAINTS VERSUS THE CAPABILITIES AND RESOURCES

Specify constraints, capabilities, resources, claimant groups

After the problem has been carefully defined and analyzed, the next step is to look at the constraints, capabilities, and resources that are available to the decision maker. Resources which will help one to make an adequate decision should not be stated in general terms but should be tied directly to specific goals and subgoals. Resources may include financial support, manpower, equipment, facilities, and technical and research assistance from other departments or units within the organization as well as those outside the organization.

It is important to list the constraints that may affect the decision making process. The nature of the constraints will affect the approach to the problem. For example, if financial constraints are of highest importance, then certain approaches to the problem may not be applicable. If a ward unit in a hospital is understaffed and each staff member must assume a range of responsibilities in order to offer the necessary patient care services, then it may be inappropriate to use a teamwork approach in solving a given patient care problem.

When analyzing the constraints, capabilities, and resources, it is also important to identify the interests that are involved in the decision since the ultimate impact of the decision will affect various persons and groups. In order to minimize the possibility of unanticipated consequences to the decision action, it is essential to ascertain which interests are important to the decision problem and which may be safely disregarded.

In each decision problem, the nurse leader must identify the multiple interests and make a reasoned judgment about the relative urgencies of these. At times it may be difficult to estimate the impact of decisions on various interest groups because it is difficult to determine in advance the meanings and values that others might place on the decision consequences. It is particularly difficult to estimate how others will view the impact of the decision on their own interests. At this stage, meetings and fact gathering activities can elicit probable impact. It is important to involve nurses at the unit level as well as middle (nursing supervisors) and top management (directors of nursing) levels early in the decision making process.

A decision will produce change. Such change may create fears and anxieties and produce resistance and hostilities. This resistance may seem irrational and unrelated to the actual benefit of the changes but must be anticipated. Resistance to change can be minimized by adequate communication, by involving all pertinent parties in decision making, and by having a systematic rationale for decisions that are made.

In considering all levels of nurses and other health care personnel before determining an approach to the solution of a problem, the decision maker can gain understanding of how various persons or groups will react to the particular course of action selected. For example, a hospital organization or institution may have impact on many groups, such as medical staff members, visiting physicians, nurses of various professional and technical levels, semiprofessionals, unskilled workers, hospital administrators, trustees, donors, fund raising groups, and volunteers. Other groups may include categories of actual and potential users, governmental agencies, medical insurance firms, professional societies, and community and political groups. These groups, any of whose interests may be affected by a decision, are called "claimant groups."[3]

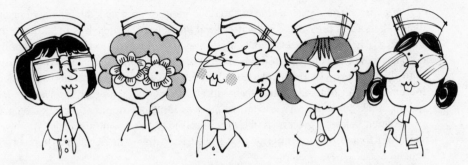

Fig. 3-3. Analyzing one's own approach is difficult since it forces examination of the lenses through which a situation is perceived.

STEP 4: SPECIFYING AN APPROACH TO SOLVING THE PROBLEM

Specify approach to problem solution

The next step in the problem solving process is to carefully define a framework for problem solution. For nurses, this involves defining the assumptions or beliefs that they hold relative to professional nursing as they care for patients and their families. For example, a psychiatric nurse may view a particular patient care problem within the framework of behavior modification. Reinforcement procedures might be used to assist the patient to resolve the problem. On the other hand, if nurses work from a gestalt therapy viewpoint, they will seek those alternatives which will enable the patient to develop a solution from his own awareness of internal and external environmental variables. It is important to note that there are various approaches and assumptions underlying problem solving.* This concept allows a different approach to be considered if a selected course of action is ineffective in solving the problem. If an approach is not specified, the decision maker is lured into the trap of viewing the approach selected as the only conceivable one. Analysis of one's own approach can be difficult since it forces one to examine the lenses, as it were, through which the entire situation is perceived.

The aproach to a problem also indicates which type of decision procedure the nurse will utilize. Will the problem be considered as singular or complex? Most complex personal and managerial decisions involve a sequence of subdecisions. For example, a young woman who graduates from a baccalaureate nursing program may decide from among many different alternatives: go to graduate school; get married; become a member of the armed services; take a job in a local hospital; or go to Europe. If graduate education is chosen, then the next step is to choose a university to attend. A nursing program must be selected and application for admission must be submitted. An unhappily married woman may seek counseling, go to work, choose to separate or to divorce, or seek some other solution. If counseling is chosen, a marriage counselor is selected. The counselor may provide a strategy by which the client may adjust or change the situation. This may involve counseling with the husband or other members of the family. A number of decisions will be made before the problem is resolved.

---

*Selecting a professional approach to problem solving requires a broad background of theory upon which the nurse can draw and a certain open-mindedness regarding the possible relevancy of any or all of them. When the decision maker knows of only one approach, the natural tendency is to promote that "pet" viewpoint, regardless of variables existent in the presenting problem.

An approach to decision making may be focused on a specific objective or on immediate relief of the pressures. The latter kind of decision approach is to "put out the brush fires first": it has also been called the "muddling through" type.[4] In this approach the decision maker directs his attention to relief of the immediate pressure without attempting to deal with all the issues involved in the problem situation. Decisions are made in small increments and objectives are given different priorities along the decision making sequence. Now pressures are created when oversights occur and other objectives are given precedence before a present problem is resolved. Nurses who use this type of approach may find their time and energy so diffused that they can never rid themselves of any problem.

If decision makers search for the first acceptable workable solution they can find, they are using what is called the "satisficing approach."[6] This simply means that the decision maker must quickly settle upon the most satisfactory solution to the problem. If the decision involves an emergency in which delay would be costly, then a satisficing approach may be possible.* If nurses are experienced, skillful, and creative in making decisions and taking actions, they may find the best solution on the first attempt. However, if the situation is not an emergency situation, the satisficing approach degenerates to a trial and error method. A nurse who utilizes this approach is vulnerable; others may later uncover a better solution that may cause the nurse to lose the trust and respect of peers.

The nature of some problems may require a decision that cannot be reanalyzed or remade at a later date without considerable difficulty. A problem of this type requires a different approach to problem solving, the "optimizing approach." The decision maker attempts to find the best possible alternative course of action, or to find the alternative which is best among those available. This approach requires more planning and effort in analyzing the value of the alternatives generated. It generally takes more time than the satisficing approach.

Some decisions have to be made without trial and error experimentation or with no testing of the end result. Examples of this type are policy decisions, which once made are difficult to retract, even if the resulting effects may not be exactly what were intended. This is particularly true of governmental decisions that involve establishment or disestablishment of large agencies or procedures. These are known as *open-loop* decisions because when the process is represented by a model, the feedback loop does not allow the results to be recirculated through the decision process and reevaluated. A cybernetic *closed-loop* procedure, on the other hand, allows information feedback which permits comparison of the decision results with objectives and criteria that were specified earlier in the sequence. Open-loop processes apply when decisions are of great moment and are irreversible. In the actual working through of such decisions, considerable attention should be paid to information gathering and analysis of alternative solutions. If, by contrast, the results of a decision will be easily reversed and if the action can be rescinded without considerable cost, then a close-loop decision making approach is probably more appropriate.

An example of an open-loop process is the establishment of a national health care insurance program. Once a major law is passed and all the machinery is set into motion, trial and error methods have no place. Extensive analysis of alternative proposals must

---

*In a crisis situation a satisficing approach may serve the purpose of momentarily decreasing anxiety and panic so that the decision maker can begin to perceive the overall dimensions of a situation and then proceed more deliberately.

be carried out before any one plan can be selected and enacted. Once chosen, correction of the policy would be inordinately expensive and complicated.

An example of a closed-loop model might be the selection of a head nurse for a pediatrics ward. Perhaps the nursing supervisor realizes that the present head nurse will be leaving to be married within a few months. The supervisor may have a good rationale for promoting an assistant head nurse of the ward to fill the position. Recruitment procedures may exist which permit her to do this. Extensive recruitment and interviewing procedures would be unnecessary and wasteful in this situation.

STEP 5: STATING SPECIFIC DECISION OBJECTIVES AND PERFORMANCE CRITERIA

State
behavioral
objectives
and
performance
criteria

This step involves the statement of behavioral or performance objectives for the decision action. Nurses must articulate precisely what they want the decision to accomplish. Decision objectives are statements of expected outcomes which should be phrased in observable performance terms.

The question of trade-offs is important here. The decision maker must weigh the expenditure of the limited resources in implementing the decision with the expected outcomes of the decision action. All objectives listed will assert some influence on the course of action that is selected. It is therefore important that decision objectives be listed in order of priority and classified according to whether they are critical or noncritical. *Critical objectives* set limits that cannot be violated by any of the generated alternatives. If the amount of money available is only $200,000, a manager would be wasting time to consider an alternative that would cost $400,000. Critical objectives must also be specified if the results are to be effective. For example, in a patient care situation, a critical objective may be to alleviate a patient's pain. Therefore, any alternative which does not alleviate the pain is not acceptable.

Desired but *noncritical objectives* are usually concerned with advantage and disadvantage as perceived from the decision maker's value system. If nurses can distinguish between objectives which *are* critical and those which they feel are desirable only, they will be less likely to select alternatives which represent their own value system and which might eventually prove unsatisfactory from the viewpoint of the patient's need and value systems. Focusing on the critical objectives at the outset can eliminte ineffective alternatives and enable the nurse to be more efficient and effective in the decision making process.

STEP 6: GENERATING AND LISTING ALTERNATIVE SOLUTIONS

List
alternative
solutions
1. _____
2. _____
3. _____
4. _____
5. _____
6. _____
7. _____

Once the goals to be achieved have been listed, the approach specified, and critical from noncritical decision criteria differentiated, alternative solutions can be generated and listed. Alternatives are generated through applying skills of information processing and creativity. Experiences, knowledge, and relevant information and facts need to be synthesized. If a group is to be used to generate alternatives, brainstorming and other group process techniques are useful.* Proper inquiry behavior includes the ability to search for, categorize, and utilize information. Capabilities, resources, and

---

*In generating alternatives nurses could involve consumers. Although the patient's notions might not fit certain constraints and criteria, they might be novel and useful if modified and they certainly will be in line with his perceptions of his needs.

constraints of the organization must all be considered in order to evaluate whether an alternative is acceptable or will be ineffective.

Generating plausible alternatives requires a careful search for specific action which will perform a precise function. The more systematically nurses use standards in the search, the more efficiently they will be able to move through a number of possibilities to find the best range of the actions. Some alternatives may appear ready-made; but, while obvious, these may not be the best ones available. Frequently alternatives may have to be invented by combining a number of ideas.

There are several ways for developing suitable alternatives, a few of which are: (1) recalling past experience; (2) obtaining ideas and expertise of group members; (3) relying on the advice or recommendations of outside qualified experts; (4) seeking the advice and expertise of colleagues or other members of the organization; and (5) forming a committee or a task force to brainstorm and use ideas of group members. Management appears to be moving in the direction of using task forces and the principles of participative management in an effort to bring about change and to use resources within the organization.

STEP 7: ANALYZING THE OPTIONS

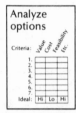

To evaluate alternative solutions that have been proposed, the alternative must be tested against the behavioral objectives stated earlier (Step 5). Such evaluation may be precise or may be estimated. The procedure entails testing each alternative against each critical objective. When an alternative fails to meet the standard of the critical objectives, the decision maker can discard that alternative. This procedure will eventually screen out the low-value, high-cost, high-risk alternatives. For some criteria such as cost, it is usually important to set maximum limits that cannot be exceeded.

Certain numerical scoring procedures can be used to speed up the analysis of alternatives. Using numbers to analyze alternatives can make the decision making process easier. The numbers serve to record the judgments made by the decision maker, and enable the decision maker to reanalyze the judgments if necessary. A numerical ordering also makes it possible to deal systematically with a number of judgments without losing sight of the goals and specific performance objectives.

Chapter 5 describes several types of criteria that can be used to screen the options or alternative solutions. For example, gain-loss tables can be constructed which will indicate the relative gain versus the possible losses if a certain alternative is selected. Another method is to consider the absolute cost as well as the relative cost of a particular alternative. This type of decision confronts many housewives when they have the opportunity to purchase a large amount of some commodity for a lower unit price. For example, a case of dry cereal may not be a good investment for certain families even though the cost per box is far below the cost of the item if purchased separately. The absolute cost for a small urban family would exceed that which would normally be expended for a perishable item. Certain circumstances, however, can be significant to the decision: if the housewife and her husband live on a farm with twelve children and three hired hands, the absolute cost may be seen as relatively small.

Another approach is to consider undesirable consequences and side effects. This approach is frequently used by physicians in prescribing drugs for patients, or by managers of organizations who recognize the importance of maintaining human relations.

STEP 8: CHOOSING THE BEST ALTERNATIVE BY APPLYING DECISION RULES

Choose:
apply
decision
rules
A. _____
B. _____
C. _____
D. _____

Once the preliminary steps have been taken, the alternative which receives the highest score on the performance objectives would normally be considered as the best course of action. But suppose there is a tie between alternatives. Or suppose there were some underlying feelings that told the nurse that the choice receiving the highest rating was not the best of alternatives. Action taken at this point might create problems that could become more serious than the original problem. Therefore, decision rules must be applied.

Developing rules for identifying the best alternative among those generated requires the decision maker to refer back to the approach and assumptions. By so doing, decision rules can become an index by which high ranking alternatives can be compared for desirability.

Decision rules are based upon the approach selected for problem solution and on the overall purposes which have been specified. For example, suppose the stated approach to a patient care problem was "patient-centered" and an overall purpose of nursing was "to involve the patient in decisions about his health care" and "to assist him to function independently." Acceptable alternatives should give the patient the opportunity to make choices. This then becomes a decision rule. Alternatives that do not allow the patient to make this choice, even though scoring high on the decision criteria, should not be selected.

Common sources of decision rules are the policies and regulations of the institution in which one is working. Although an alternative might meet all of the criteria established for its acceptability, if the policy manual will not allow such an action, that alternative obviously should not be chosen (unless the nurse can successfully challenge the stated policy). But such action takes time, data, and clout—resources that may not be available.

STEP 9: CONTROL AND IMPLEMENTATION OF DECISION ACTION

Control
and
implement
decisions

The final step in the problem solving process is highly relevant to the entire procedure. In the first part of this step the decision maker attempts to control the effects of final decisions by means of control measures.* This must be done before taking actions so that adverse consequences can be presented.

Certain known procedures can effectively help the decision maker control and implement a decision. First, reporting procedures should be established so that the progress of a decision action can be compared against the schedule for putting it into effect. Second, a follow-up on any directives to staff members should be undertaken to determine if the directives have been properly received and understood. Third, the person who is to be responsible for carrying out the directives should be designated and the responsibilities and tasks clearly defined. Fourth, a warning system should be established to indicate as early as possible that the decision is headed for difficulties. Fifth, specific reporting dates should be set so that the action being taken can be systematically evaluated.

---

*The word control here does not indicate arbitrary or authoritarian methods; it refers to the manager's ability to direct and monitor a process. A critical component of control is feedback. The manager must be able to obtain relevant information regarding the status of a decision action. Control is a form of continuous and ongoing evaluation.

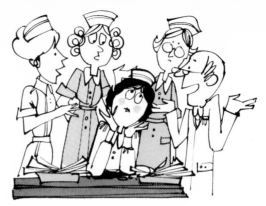

Fig. 3-4. A warning system should be established to indicate as early as possible that the decision is headed for difficulties.

STEP 10: EVALUATING THE EFFECTIVENESS OF A DECISION ACT

Evaluate effectiveness of action

Results

Correction or supplementation

After the environment in which the decision will operate has been controlled and the decision action implemented, a procedure is needed for analyzing the effectiveness of the selected course of action. Formal evaluation consists of comparing the observable performance results of a decision with standards that have been determined earlier. Negative feedback in the evaluation process indicates that the decision action taken did not solve the problem and that the decision was ineffective. Corrective or supplementary action can then be taken. The decision can be recycled through the problem solving sequence, beginning at any point where a difficulty is evident. Positive feedback indicates that the proper action was taken.

Effective problem solvers and decision makers use systematic procedures. Nurses working in a variety of situations can become effective managers if they adopt a systematic approach to the problems they face. In the complex health care delivery systems of today, the nurse cannot base decisions on intuition. As Peter Drucker has said:

> Most managers know that they need better tools. Most have learned by bitter experience that intuition is unreliable, if not downright treacherous, if used as the only basis for decision.[*]

---

[*] From Drucker, P. F.: Management: tasks, responsibilities, practices, New York, 1973, Harper & Row, Publishers, p. 507.

REFERENCES

1. Drucker, P. F.: Management: tasks, responsibilities, practices, New York, 1973, Harper & Row, Publishers.
2. Drucker, P. F.: The effective executive, New York, 1967, Harper & Row, Publishers.
3. Easton, A.: Claimantship versus membership as organizational constructs, J. Human Relations **17:**71-76, 1969.
4. Lindblom, C. E.: The science of muddling through, Public Administration Review **19:** 79-88, 1959.
5. Simon, H. A.: Models of man, New York, 1957, John Wiley & Sons, Inc.
6. Simon, H. A.: The new science of management decision, New York, 1960, Harper & Row, Publishers.

SUGGESTED READINGS

Daubenmire, J. M., and King, I. M.: Nursing process models: a systems approach, Nurs. Outlook **21:**512-517, 1973.

Leininger, M.: An open health care system model, Nurs. Outlook **21:**171-175, 1973.

Newell, A., and Simon, H. S.: Human problem solving, Englewood Cliffs, N. J., 1972, Prentice-Hall, Inc.

Odiorne, G. S.: Management decisions by objectives, Englewood Cliffs, N. J., 1969, Prentice-Hall, Inc.

The secret to success is constancy to purpose.

B. DISRAELI

Define
overall
needs,
purposes,
goals

4 DEFINING OVERALL NEEDS, PURPOSES, AND GOALS

The problem solving process begins with a felt need—a perception of the need for change. A felt need may be an urge for improving a situation that has certain inadequacies; or it may be an intense dissatisfaction with the entire situation and a desire to bring about drastic changes.

Motivation for change can grow from one person's perception of a need. This person might be a nurse in a middle management position such as a head nurse. Change can also be imposed within organizations by top management. The bedside nurse also senses the need for change and begins to solve problems in direct patient care. Ultimately someone has to feel pressure for a change in the status quo and then take action. There is nothing mysterious about why the need for change is felt in most cases. Effective decision makers can usually identify these situations and respond appropriately. It is the responses of decision makers that we are about to examine.

The perception of a need for change indicates that the system's performance differs from an expectation. Expectations are based upon objectives from which standards are derived. Although objectives are related to and similar to goals and standards, they are not exactly the same. A consideration of how these terms are related to problem solving and how they differ may clarify distinctions between these concepts.

A review of the literature which describes managerial decision making and problem solving indicates that there is general agreement that purposes, goals, and objectives should be stated clearly before attempting to solve a given problem. These terms (purposes, goals, and objectives) tend to be used interchangeably. In practice, it is helpful to make a distinction between these terms so that the various steps in the problem solving/decision making sequence become clear and useful in the overall procedure.

PURPOSES

Purposes are the overall ends toward which organizations, departments, units, groups, or individuals strive. Purposes can be controlled only in a limited way. A number of external forces have influence over purposes. Needs provide the basis of purposes. There is a similarity in needs whether they come from an individual or from a large organization.

For example, one may think of the individual or organization as constantly growing, which means that the needs and purposes are continually changing in number and in kind. This is sometimes referred to as a change in need level. With this process of change in mind, it becomes apparent that over a period of time the needs of a person will be interrelated and changing. Although such a concept may appear paradoxical at first, it can be understood when examined within the context of experiences. Individuals function at several need levels in the process of becoming adults.

The purpose of becoming

A purpose which is shared by all humans and organizations is that of *becoming*. Becoming is growth toward ultimate potential and maturity. Maslow called this purpose "self actualization." An examination of the age continuum from birth to death indicates a steady advancement or movement toward maturity in the kinds of needs experiences. This concept is often described as personal growth toward self-actualization. Since self-actualization is the most complete state of development, growth is characterized by flexibility (the opposite of rigidity) in the person or organization. Flexibility includes the ability to adapt successfully to the environment, and represents an element that may not be reached by everyone.

TYPES OF NEEDS

Nurses must be aware of the need levels of their patients in order to direct and administer patient care. Being concerned with what recent postoperative patients would like for lunch the next day may not be as important in meeting their needs as seeing that their supine position induces a feeling of comfort and aids circulatory processes and attitude.

Maslow's study of human needs and their influence on behavior provides a comprehensive approach for looking at needs.[4] Maslow presents five major categories of human needs that exist in a hierarchy (see Fig. 4-2). The concept of homeostasis models the origin of these needs. When equilibrium or optimum balance within our bodies is disturbed, the body automatically seeks a coordinated response to compensate for the element that is lacking, or to compensate for environmental changes.

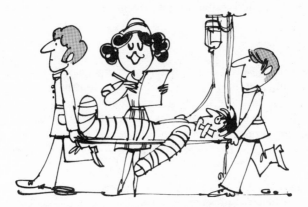

Fig. 4-1. What would you like for lunch tomorrow?

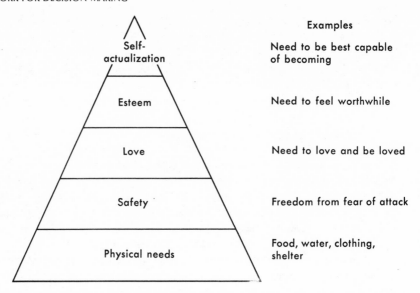

Fig. 4-2. Maslow's need hierarchy.

Physiological needs

The physiological needs, or needs of the body, are the most elementary needs in Maslow's hierarchy. All living animals experience these needs and are motivated to satisfy urges such as hunger, thirst, fatigue, sexual desire, and others. A person who is suffering from hunger will not be free to satisfy other higher needs until the hunger need is met. Being deprived of food can motivate a person to direct all actions toward obtaining food. A need for food may overshadow needs for safety or self-esteem.

The Maslow hierarchy illustrates that the whole man experiences a need. For example, the effects of hunger are not confined to the digestive system. Imbalances in various parts of the body will occur. A person may become irritable and have difficulty concentrating. If a person is extremely hungry, he may be willing to put himself in jeopardy by stealing in order to obtain food. The verbal expression of this need shows that the totality of the feeling—"I am hungry"—is a different statement from saying "My stomach is hungry." By having something to eat, a person satisfies this need, is no longer motivated by it, and is then able to become aware of other types of needs.

Safety needs

According to Maslow, when a physiological need is satisfied, a person's concern will turn to seeking safety. At one time, safety may have meant staying downwind of tigers. Today, safety may mean seeking an environment in which one is safe from physical or emotional assaults,* or safe from catastrophic forces such as earthquakes or tornadoes.

The people who want and seek safety frequently depend on help from others, such as police protection. Children also want to feel safe and to live in an environment that is orderly and predictable. They show a preference for regularity, routine, and assurance

---

*An emotional assault can cause fear. Defensive behavior in interpersonal relations is calculated to keep us safe from embarrassment, feelings of inadequacy, or rejection. The common human fear of new situations and new people stems from this second level of safety needs.

that should harm come their parents will protect them. Safety needs of adults may be as acute as those of children, but in our society adults learn to repress signs of these concerns.

Love needs

When the physiological and safety needs are met, a person may experience a desire for love and affection. A person who is lonely may have an overwhelming need for love and affection. This need may be felt as wanting to have friends, a family, or a boyfriend or girlfriend. The intensity of this drive is no less than that experienced by the hungry man in search of food. Many of the severe neuroses that exist are known to come from a deep sense of not being loved or of not belonging. Feelings of not being loved or of not belonging are not the same as the need for sex. Belongingness needs are a part of a sexual impulse, but unlike sexual behavior they are not basically physiological.

Esteem needs

Progressing through Maslow's hierarchy presented in Fig. 4-2, the next need is for esteem, which represents a variety of needs with common characteristics. These needs can be classified into two groups. The first of these needs includes a need to feel independent, or to feel free. A sense of feeling capable, strong, and confident characterizes these needs. A second group of needs includes the social complement of inner confidence. Recognition from others, prestige, and status are representative of this group. People whose esteem needs are satisfied feel that what they are and what they do are important to the world. Maslow points out that the soundest basis for esteem is well-deserved respect from others rather than praise that may not be justified.

Studies of esteem indicate that jobs which individuals find satisfying are those which allow them to increase their knowledge and skills. When an individual grows in competence and expertise, and when these qualities are demonstrated, fellow workers tend to increase their trust and respect for the person.

Self-actualization

Some individuals whose esteem needs and lower needs in the hierarchy are satisfied may continue to experience deep-felt discontent. Maslow refers to this final craving as the need for self-actualization—the desire to become all that one is capable of becoming and to feel that one is doing what is right for him. If this need is not met in a life role, in a job or profession, the need may be satisfied through leisure activities. The degree to which a person is able to reach his capabilities is important to feelings of maturity and self-actualization.

Maslow's need hierarchy is a useful concept but cannot be rigidly applied to everyone. There are probably people whose need for recognition far outweighs the need for love. For example, an artist's need for self-fulfillment may be more urgent than some of his more basic needs.

The needs of a person with a particular personality type may be an outcome of how the personality developed. If a person's early years were devoid of love and affection, he may eventually find his need for giving and receiving love relatively unimportant. To a person who has never had the experience of hunger, the need for food may seem inconsequential.

From the conceptual framework of Maslow's hierarchy, it might be assumed that a need cannot be felt until those needs which appear at the lower levels in the hierarchy have been totally satisfied. A more accurate assumption is that all basic needs are only partially satisfied. There is a great deal of overlap and shifting in a person's hierarchy of needs.

Perhaps behavior can best be understood as a continual effort to reduce the pressure caused by needs. Often this behavior is oriented to some goal which is also a product of a felt need.

TYPES OF PURPOSES BASED UPON NEEDS

Purposes are drives that are based on needs. They are not limited to the animal world. Overall purposes of organizations or systems can also be explained in terms of Maslow's hierarchy of needs.[2] The list of needs and their related purposes when applied within the broadest context of an organization or system can be illustrated as follows:

Level One—Survival: These purposes refer to the very existence of the organization or system.

Level Two—Stability: These purposes reflect a need for order and predictability in operation.

Level Three—Belongingness: Purposes at this level refer to the image a system or an organization projects and the degree to which the group members identify.

Level Four—Esteem and status needs: These needs reflect the ability or the desire of the organization to differentiate and develop its unique position.

Level Five—Self-actualization: These purposes indicate that the organization is secure and willing to take risks. They demonstrate a willingness to experiment. Creativity is often evident when needs are being met at this level.

An organization or system cannot have complete control over the purpose level at which it operates. This level is often a function of the influence and control exercised by various claimant groups and clients. For example, a hospital might aspire to operate above the survival level, but constraints such as financial problems may keep the organization at a low purpose level.

All levels of needs may be evident in an organization. A hospital provides an example: Level One needs would be manifested in budgets and building plans; Level Two needs would be reflected in the organization of personnel to permit effective functioning; Level Three needs produce a desire for the community to accept the hospital and patronize it and the desire for staff to work in it; Level Four needs are reflected in the desire to become accredited by the American Hospital Association and to be respected by other hospitals and health care facilities; and Level Five needs are displayed in the development of new services to meet community health needs, expansion of services, and experimental programs in staffing and administration.

GOALS

Goals are statements of intent or outcomes. Goal statements derive from purposes, which in turn derive from needs. Goals are usually general in nature and provide bases for operating guidelines for those who work within an organization. Goal statements themselves are not quantifiable—they cannot be measured. They are usually generalizations that are operant to *everyone whom they affect* until performance objectives are identified.

Although a goal may be perceived as an abstraction, it describes a particular outcome. A goal statement does not describe the process necessary to reach the goal. Goal statements which imply something about how the goal is to be achieved require revision and

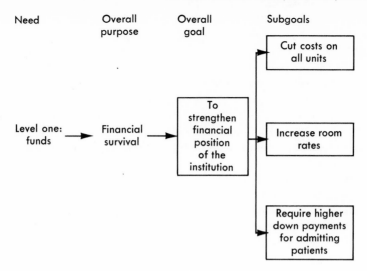

Fig. 4-3. Relationship between needs, purposes, and goals in a hospital having basic financial needs.

refinement. Stating goals precisely is a difficult undertaking. Probably the most common fault with goal statements is that they try to do more than they need to do. A goal should indicate the end product—the outcome. Fig. 4-3 illustrates the relationship between needs, purposes, and goals.

Most organizations have multiple goals. When the goals are derived from the purposes and are reasonable and congruent with each other, they can serve as guidelines for behavior. Goals can serve to discourage deviant behavior as well as be a basis for rewarding appropriate behavior. Most goals appear to be congruent as long as they are talked about in general terms. For example, a university teaching hospital may have the following goals: (1) to provide quality patient care; (2) to provide and expand professional health education; and (3) to promote and apply health science knowledge to health problems through research and creative work.

All of these goals may appear to be worthwhile and congruent. But when the goals are operationalized (that is, described in terms of observable performance) they may appear less congruent. For example, a hospital may allow the patient to make decisions about his own health care procedures. He may be permitted to refuse treatment and sign himself out of the hospital even though this may have adverse consequences in terms of his health status and in terms of the goals of the hospital. Thus, general health care goals are not always compatible with the need level or goals of individual patients at any given time.

Goals enable persons within organizations to have general guidelines against which they can judge specific actions. If certain members of a team consistently behave in a manner which is contrary to stated goals, the goals can be useful in dealing with undesirable behavior. The impersonal quality of a stated goal can be a valid and tactful way of presenting problems to offenders, or of rewarding individuals for their achievements.

OBJECTIVES

Objectives, unlike goals, are quantifiable. They are specific statements that refer to observable behaviors. Objectives should contribute to goals and be derived from the goal statement. For example, one of the goals of the hospital discussed earlier is to provide quality health care. This goal could be quantified and explicated by a nursing service department as follows: to provide the patient with continuity of care through extending patient care services to the home or to other care settings if indicated.

Nurses must be careful as they deal with problems and work with behavioral objectives that they do not lose sight of the overall purposes and goals of the health care organization. If the overall purposes and goals are overlooked, external forces may exert pressure to reduce the purpose level (need level) at which the organization is operating. For example, a community health care clinic might become so involved in providing direct patient care that it fails to develop the research purposes for which it was originally funded and thus loses government support and funding. Social scientists refer to this phenomenon of overly focusing on objectives without relating them to purposes and goals as "goal displacement."

Since objectives are designed to be quantifiable, they must be stated in terms which allow them to be measured. If objectives are specific, observable, and measurable, they should become the major focus of nursing in health care settings. Objectives can be used to demonstrate to outside investigators such as accrediting agencies that something is being done and that the organization knows how effectively it is being done.

BEHAVIORAL OBJECTIVES LEAD TO PERFORMANCE CRITERIA

Stating objectives in behavioral terms means that objectives can be measured by reference to observable behavior. Well-stated behavioral objectives yield performance criteria, the specific measurement categories (discussed in Chapter 10). Performance criteria become the basis for analyzing decision alternatives in the decision making process. It is therefore extremely important that performance criteria are based on objectives which have been clearly delineated at an earlier stage in the process. If this has not been done, it will be difficult to see the relationship of behavioral objectives to other objectives.

Furthermore, objectives must be quantifiable. This condition can be met if the objectives are stated in behavioral or performance terms. Evaluators can look at the actions or behavior of those who are being assessed and determine whether or not the individual is meeting the objective. Goals, on the other hand, are effective for public relations purposes, and for providing guidelines against which to compare objectives.

The subject of behavioral objectives is receiving widespread attention in nursing. Nurses are being exposed to the concept of accountability through conferences and numerous meetings sponsored by professional organizations. Accountability, which places a high value on the judgmental skills of the nurse, provides further impetus for stating objectives in behavioral terms.

Fig. 4-4 summarizes the relationships between needs, purposes, goals, behavioral objectives, and performance criteria. The progression is from the felt needs and drives, to more narrowly articulated statements of goals and objectives, to the very specific criteria which are used to measure performance.

MAJOR CATEGORIES OF GOALS AND OBJECTIVES

Goals and objectives fall primarily into three major categories: those concerned with content or product, those concerned with attitude and other affective or emotional variables, and those concerned with the psychomotor performance skills. Objectives concerned with content and product are called *cognitive,* and refer to knowledge, thinking, and other intellectual processes. The second category of goals and objectives refers to

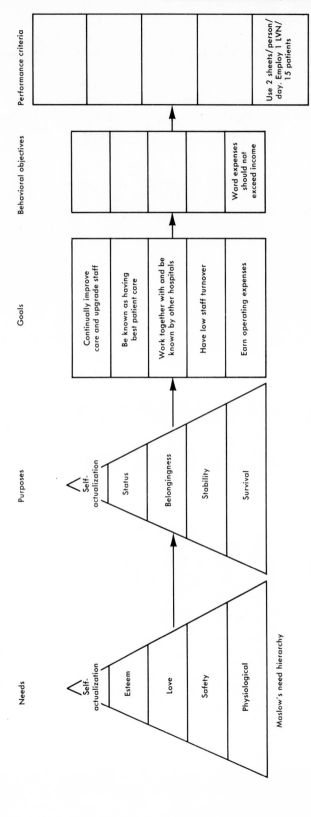

Fig. 4-4. Relationship of needs, purposes, goals, behavioral objectives, and performance criteria using a hospital example.

feelings, emotions, and attitudes toward a product or process; these are called the *affective* goals. The third category, which is very important to nursing, has been identified by psychologists as the *psychomotor* domain. This category of objectives is concerned with physiological characteristics and physical capabilities of a person.

The differences between these three types of goals are quite marked: (1) cognitive goals and objectives emphasize intellectual tasks and knowledge acquisition; (2) affective objectives emphasize a feeling, tone, or emotion; and (3) psychomotor goals emphasize capabilities and performance of tasks.

GOAL ANALYSIS

The process of goal analysis is essentially the process of separating abstractions from performance statements.[3] As mentioned earlier, a goal should describe an outcome rather than a process. The decision maker who keeps this in mind is less likely to become bogged down with the philosophical problem of means and ends. It is important to specify a goal that is an outcome statement so that at a later stage behavioral objectives and performance criteria can be determined. The performance criteria will be those that are used to analyze the alternative solutions to a problem. One test to determine whether a goal is a statement of an outcome is fairly simple: ask if there is a single act that someone might perform that will identify whether or not the goal has been achieved. To write a goal that lends itself to this test is difficult but extremely critical.

If a goal refers to some internal process then it must be translated into some observable output; another term for these observable outputs is "indicator behaviors." These behaviors indicate whether or not the behavior that is being encouraged has occurred.

SETTING UP PRIORITIES

To enable the decision maker to solve a problem, it is important that objectives of an organization or a patient care plan be rank ordered in importance. This is the first step in determining priorities. Objectives and goals should be rank ordered in two categories: (1) those that are critical or absolutely essential to the welfare or purposes of the organization or person at the time, and (2) those that are nonessential but desired goals of the organization.[1]

Every decision maker should appreciate the importance of the organization's goals and objectives. These goals and objectives will generate the criteria which will help determine whether the system is effective or not. Indeed, performance review and accountability of an individual within an organization are integral parts of the organization's goals and objectives. Therefore objectives become the basis for activity in an organization. If objectives are not clearly stated and listed in order of priority, an organization may fail to achieve its overall aims and purposes.

REFERENCES

1. Kepner, C. H., and Tregoe, B. B.: The rational manager, New York, 1965, McGraw-Hill Book Co.
2. Lippitt, G. L., and Schmidt, W. H.: Crises in a developing organization, Harvard Business Review **45:**102-112, 1967.
3. Mager, R. F.: Goal analysis, Belmont, Calif., 1972, Fearon Publishers.
4. Maslow, A.: Motivation and personality, New York, 1954, Harper & Row, Publishers.

SUGGESTED READINGS

Cannon, W. G.: Wisdom of the body, New York, 1932, Norton.
Gross, B. M.: What are your organization's objectives? A general systems approach to planning, Human Relations **43:**205-211, 1964.
Hughes, C. L.: Goal setting: key to individual and organizational effectiveness, New York, 1965, American Management Association.
Palmer, J.: JONA refresher—management by objectives, J. Nurs. Admin. **3:**55-60, 1973.

Yedvab, J. O.: Consumer's role in defining goals,
structures, and services, Hosp. Prog. **55:**56-60,
1974.
Young, P. T.: The experimental analysis of appetite, Psychol. Bull. **38:**129-164, 1941.
Young, P. T.: Appetite, palatability and feeding
habit; a critical review, Psychol. Bull. **45:**289-
320, 1948.

*Basic to the problem-solving process is the fact that it starts
from motivation–the feeling held by an individual or a group of
individuals that some state of affairs is unsatisfactory.*

G. L. LIPPITT*

5 DIAGNOSING A PROBLEM

RECOGNIZING A PROBLEM

When needs, purposes, and the overall goals have been defined and ranked in order
of importance, the next step is to identify problems and to set priorities for resolving them.
Although determination of priorities often appears to be a difficult task, it is simplified
when the goals have been rank-ordered. For example, if a major goal of nursing service
in a particular hospital is to provide quality patient-centered care, problems related to
housekeeping will have a low priority or perhaps be dispensed with and delegated to the
ward manager. A nurse who chooses to become involved in such housekeeping problems
is delaying the task of dealing with problems that are more directly related to meeting
the needs of patients. Actions centered on nonnursing functions create an atmosphere
of continuous unresolved patient-care problems.

Two conditions must exist before a discrepancy is classified as a problem. First, someone needs to feel that there is a difference or discrepancy between expected performance
and actual performance. If a person's standards are low, then few things will be seen as
problems. On the other hand, if a person has extremely high standards, more problems
are likely to be seen. Some health care situations require higher standards than others.
In such situations, problems will arise more frequently because there are more opportunities for discrepancies or deviations to occur.

The second condition that is necessary before a discrepancy can be classified as a
problem is that someone must want to find the cause of what is wrong and seek to correct
it. Problems related to performance will not be identified unless there is concern expressed for discrepancies between observed performance and performance standards.

STEP 2: DEFINING THE PROBLEM

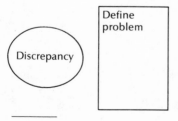

Problem analysis begins with the individual's store of
relevant information about the standards that have been
set and the actual performances that have been observed.
The next step is to identify those things that have gone
wrong and to hypothesize or try to determine which
things may have caused the change of behavior. Often
a nurse is confronted with a number of problems, in-

*From Lippitt, G. L.: Organizational renewal: achieving viability in a changing world, New York,
1969, Appleton-Century-Crofts, p. 153.

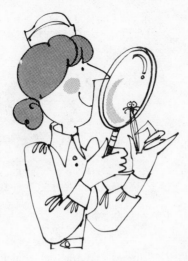

Fig. 5-1. The nurse must survey the situation and determine what is actually happening.

cluding patient care problems, managerial problems, or perhaps a combination of both. Because of the multiplicity of problems with which nurses are confronted, the rank ordering of priorities that have been established will be helpful. That is, nurses will be able to look at goals and their rank order to determine which discrepancy will be dealt with first. This assessment is an information processing period in the decision making process as well as the nursing process. The nurse must survey the situation and determine what is actually happening. In doing this, a nurse uses basic skills of observation and data recording. When a nurse has adequate knowledge of expected performance standards, discrepancies in performance can be identified and dealt with easily.

The expertise of nurses, as they become familiar with this approach to problems, may be such that they will see problems which others have overlooked. The ability to identify problems and to determine priorities can make a tremendous difference in resolving the crisis in the health care system and in bringing about change.

When surveying problems, nurses should be wary of lumping them all together. Clustering of discrepancies could produce inadequate descriptions such as "communications problem" or "morale problem." These labels are rather useless and may only produce a list of problems that have the same cause. Fuzzy thinking in identifying a problem will confuse and obscure the results.

How to describe a problem. A problem clearly and precisely described is requisite to problem solution. Problem description is based on a careful and selective information search. It is helpful to have guidelines for this search. Kepner and Tregoe[1] have developed a system for specifying problems that involves asking four critical questions:

1. *What* is the deviation (from standards) and what is the thing or object on which the deviation is observed?
2. *Where* is the deviation on the thing or object, and where are objects with the deviation observed?
3. *When* does the deviation appear on the thing or object, and when are objects with the deviation observed?
4. *How big* are the deviations, and how many objects with deviations are observed?

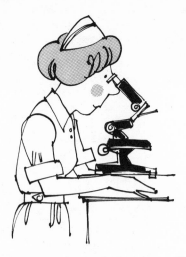

Fig. 5-2. The expertise of nurses may be such that they will see problems that others have overlooked.

They deal at length with the procedures for obtaining answers to the four questions. The process outlined has been successful in a variety of industrial settings.

By expanding the Kepner-Tregoe procedure, health care delivery problems can be defined. Five basic questions provide a framework for nurse managers to use in determining what constitutes relevant information in problem solving and how to eliminate information that is irrelevant and superficial.

A problem can be systematically specified and defined if the following five questions are asked and answered:

1. What is happening?
2. Where is it happening?
3. When is it happening?
4. What is the extent of the observed discrepancy? (How much? How many? How far?)
5. What is the nature of the happening? (Is it stable or variable?)

No other questions should be asked until these five questions are answered. Asking and answering these questions in an attempt to describe the problem may appear disarmingly simple, even mechanical. For this reason it demands disciplined thinking. The urge may be extremely strong to look for the cause of a problem immediately. Looking for the cause, however, comes later. Problem solvers can go wrong when they jump to conclusions. A favorite "why" can set the entire process off course. Watch out for statements such as: "Oh, I know why that happened," or "Well, if he hadn't done that, this never would have happened." These are typical indicators that someone is jumping to the "why," and to the cause of the problem. The problem solver must be careful to rigorously exclude assumptions, and learn to rely upon relevant factual information.

The process described sounds easy, but it demands rigorous discipline and thought. Most people find it much easier to draw a conclusion than to systematically set decision making behavior into motion.

A system for gathering data. If the problem solver is to obtain relevant facts that will help describe the problem, a system for gathering and reviewing data is necessary. It is helpful to think of the problem identification process as a cybernetic subsystem within

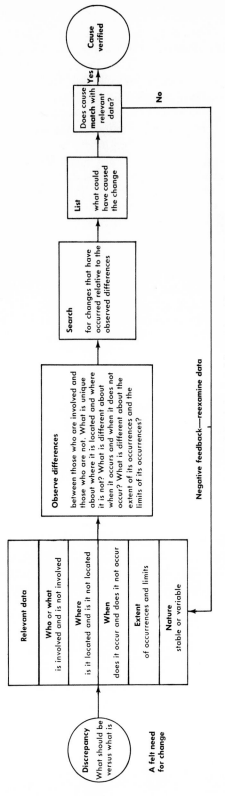

Fig. 5-3. A systems model of the problem identification process.

the problem solving process. Problem identification begins with a felt need for change as input to the system. The problem solver transforms data obtained from the problem environment into facts that answer or fail to answer the five basic questions. The system narrows down the data to possible causes, which become feedback into the system and are tested against the facts originally collected. If the feedback yields a positive match, then the problem has been identified.

To assist the nurse problem solver obtain facts that will help describe a problem, a systems format has been developed around the five questions discussed earlier. Fig. 5-3 provides a systematic guide for sorting information into useful categories for analysis. The use of a systematic framework enables the problem solver to concentrate on relevant information and to avoid collecting more data than is necessary to describe the problem. The problem solver will be less likely to jump to conclusions and go off on a wasteful search for possible causes before the relevant facts have been gathered. Without such guidelines for categorizing the facts, it is difficult to arrive at a precise description of a discrepancy.

Experience and direct observation are not always helpful in an information search and in recognizing pertinent facts. Technical know-how does not guarantee a precise description of a problem. In fact, technical experience can blind a person to the very facts that might lead to a solution. This has been demonstrated when people have pursued the irresistible "why" with the assumption: "I know what is causing the problem."

When assumptions are made about what is right and what is wrong in a situation, the assumptions then become the basis for action. How many times have you seen: expensive new equipment ordered which did not solve the problem; people fired, which did nothing to resolve a problem; new and difficult procedures introduced that were highly ineffective and almost impossible to undo once they were instituted? These examples represent a waste of time, energy, effort, and money.

A process of narrowing down. The problem solver starts by gathering facts which relate to the five critical questions described earlier. Once the facts have been gathered, comparisons and contrasts are made which will highlight areas where distinctions exist. These distinctions between the problem area and other similar areas provide clues to possible causes. Such causes are usually rooted in some change that has occurred somewhere along the line. Pinpointing the nature of that change or the direction from the desired standards (the "should" or "could be") leads directly to specifying the problem. Once the precise nature of the discrepancy can be described, it is then possible to search for possible causes. Hypotheses about the cause can be tested directly be referring back to the facts collected earlier when answering the five questions.

The problem solver need only ask: "Would this probable cause have caused *all* of the listed conditions?" A process of narrowing down will focus on the most probable cause. Then the problem solver is ready to consider the next steps in the process. The process of systematically narrowing down the data is graphically described in Fig. 5-3.

At each stage, problem solvers are concerned with fewer facts until at last they can deal with the "whys"—the possible causes. By comparing the hypothesized "whys" with the facts, problem solvers can discover the most likely cause of the problem. They are now ready to *start* to solve it.

What the problem is. The problem solver must first list those facts that precisely describe the discrepancy that has been observed. The list should include any objects or people that may have been affected by the discrepancy.

The list may be difficult to comprise in health care situations, where signs and symptoms abound and where multiple health professionals are involved. The nurse who is a problem solver must be able to sift through a morass of data to describe precisely what is happening. Guidelines are provided by the following steps and questions: (1) Determine the nature of the happening: Which patients are involved? Which personnel? (2) Where is the problem occurring? (3) Look at the timing: When is it happening? What is the range of times when it is occurring? When did it start? When did it stop? (4) Determine the extent of the discrepancy: How much deviation is there in the discrepancy from the desired or stated standards? How many things are involved? (5) Determine the stability of the discrepancy: Is the discrepancy constant or is it variable?

Using the format just described and presented in Fig. 5-3 enables the nurse to organize facts clearly and in an orderly way.

What the problem is not. Kepner and Tregoe[1] indicate that the problem analysis procedure rests on the ability of the manager to distinguish what the problem is from what it is not. By carefully describing those things or people that are closely related to the discrepancy but are not affected by it, the nurse manager can gather clues to changes that may have occurred. To make a precise problem description, it is necessary to be able to compare problem areas to those areas that are not a problem. While thinking about what the problem is not, the decision maker is forced to focus on the precise facts in a situation. If the "is nots" are carefully listed, one can easily recognize distinctions that may exist between the two sets of facts. These distinctions will give clues to the cause of the problem.

For example, when dealing with a patient care problem, the nurse would ask if the trouble was with all the patients on the ward or with just some of the patients. If the problem was noted in all the patients on that particular ward, then the next question might be "What is the most closely related group of patients where there is not trouble of this type and where you might expect to find it?" As the problem description becomes narrower, the distinction will appear sharper.

The distinction between what is and what is not. When describing a problem, it is helpful to think first about what the problem is before looking at what it is not. This will tend to keep the decision maker from jumping to conclusions or favoring one set of facts over another. After listing what the problem is not, the next step is to note any distinctions that come to mind between the group of patients that is having the problem and the group of patients that is most similar to them but is *not* having the problem.

The next question to ask is whether or not any changes have occurred in a procedure or in personnel. If so, precisely when the changes occurred needs to be determined.

What are some possible causes? After changes have been noted, the decision maker can think about possible causes. The search for a cause is basically a three-stage process: (1) the first step consists of looking at what is distinctive about the "is" data compared to the "is not" data; (2) next comes the description of changes that have taken place either prior to or during the period of time when the discrepancy has been noted. A simple or complex change may be responsible for the problem. The clues as to how the change occurred are important. These clues indicate what types of alternative solutions might be most likely to remedy the situation. (3) Finally, the search for causes requires matching the hypothesized causes with the facts that are listed. A relevant question to obtain this information and which should be formalized is: "Could this cause have yielded all these results?" If the answer is "yes," the problem solver has identified the problem.

REFERENCE

1. Kepner, C. H., and Tregoe, B. B.: The rational manager, New York, 1965, McGraw-Hill Book Co.

SUGGESTED READINGS

Lippitt, G. L.: Organizational renewal: achieving viability in a changing world, New York, 1969, Appleton-Century-Crofts.

Mager, R. F., and Pipe, P.: Analyzing performance problems, Belmont, Calif., 1970, Fearon Publishers.

McDonnel, C., Kramer, M., and Leak, A.: What would you do? Am. J. Nurs. **72:**296-301, 1972.

Problem awareness must be translated into a desire to change,
and this in turn requires a readiness and capacity to change.

G. L. LIPPITT*

Specify constraints, capabilities, resources, claimant groups

6 ANALYZING CONSTRAINTS, CAPABILITIES, AND RESOURCES

Before decision makers can develop an approach to solving a problem which has been defined, they must carefully analyze three major areas: (1) the constraints which operate upon the decision maker, upon the organization, or upon the groups that will be affected; (2) the capabilities and resources available to the decision maker or the organization; and (3) the interest groups that will be affected by the decision.

WEIGHING THE RELATIVE IMPORTANCE OF CONSTRAINTS VERSUS CAPABILITIES

Before an analysis of constraints can be performed, decision makers need to list the constraints within which they must work. Having listed such constraints, the next step is to look at capabilities. It is helpful if the decision maker regards these two lists as single phenomena being analyzed through different perspectives. Categories of constraints and capabilities which should be considered include the following:

1. Time
2. Financial support
3. Equipment and facilities
4. Interaction and assistance within the organization
5. Manpower
6. Outside assistance
7. The environment

ANALYZING THE RELATIVE STRENGTH OF CONSTRAINTS VERSUS CAPABILITIES

Force field analysis is a useful tool for analyzing constraints and capabilities. The approach was developed by the social scientist, Kurt Lewin, to determine the forces which are at work when a change is being introduced and to determine the relative strength of each of the two opposing forces.[1,2] When introducing change it is helpful to

---

*From Lippitt, G. L.: Organizational renewal: achieving viability in a changing world, New York, 1969, Appleton-Century-Crofts, p. 159.

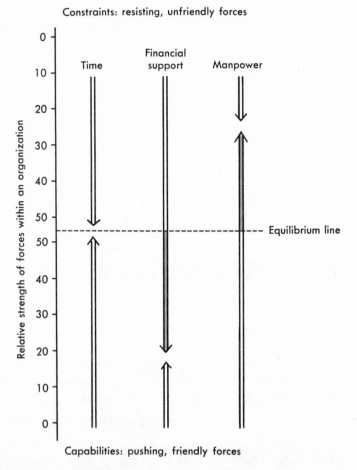

Fig. 6-1. Estimation of strength of forces affecting a potential change.

know what elements are pushing or assisting a change agent to bring about change, and what forces are restraining or working against planned change. These opposing forces provide a change agent with clues as to how to weaken the restraining forces and how to strengthen the forces that are pushing for change.

Whether a particular problem is a change problem or not, the force field analysis technique is useful in estimating the relative strength of the capabilities and constraints which affect the decision maker and which will eventually affect the outcome and impact of the decision made. After the decision maker has listed capabilities and constraints, it is easy to analyze the relative strengths and weaknesses of each of these opposing forces. Fig. 6-1 illustrates the relative strength of forces that might affect a potential decision to change. Fig. 6-2 shows how a simple profile of the constraints and capabilities can be developed from a force field analysis. Armed with such a diagram the nurse manager is better able to strategize the highest and best use of the available resources.

In analyzing capabilities and constraints, the decision maker considers the relative strength of the two types of forces. For example, the decision maker may find that time is neither a capability nor a constraint. That is, there may be adequate time to enact a decision or to begin a new program. In this case, the decision maker perceives time as

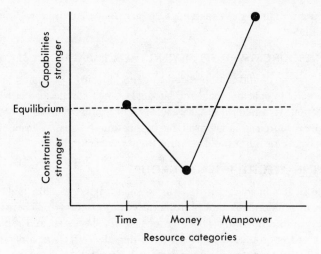

Fig. 6-2. Profile of a force field analysis.

Goals	Resources				Timing
	People	Funds	Material	Organization	

Fig. 6-3. Format for relating resources to goals and time period for which resources are allocated.

neither a capability nor a constraint, and the time factor would be rated as having equal influence.

Suppose, however, that financial support for a program is meager. In this case, the constraints would far outweigh the capabilities. Thus the decision maker would rate the constraint as a much stronger force, as presented in Fig. 6-1. Suppose that in the category of manpower there is more than adequate manpower to do a desired task and to achieve a goal. This capability would be more powerful than the constraint of not having enough manpower. The decision maker would then indicate the stronger force of capabilities on the profile sheet presented in Fig. 6-2.

At the conclusion of the force field analysis procedure, the decision maker would have a profile of capabilities and constraints for designated categories. This data would be helpful in planning strategies, and would influence the approach to the problem solution. A planning strategy might be to develop an approach that would minimize the effects of the financial constraint but would maximize the capabilities of manpower. If a nurse can develop a profile of the capabilities versus the constraints, selection of an approach will be facilitated.

IDENTIFYING RESOURCES AND SPECIFYING THEIR IMPACT OR USE

Resources should not be stated in general terms but should be specifically listed and tied directly to specific goals and subgoals. They should also be allocated within a given time period. It is helpful to take each one of the listed goals in order of priority and consider the resources that are available in meeting the goal. A format is presented in Fig. 6-3 for analyzing resources and relating them to specific goals.

IDENTIFYING THE AFFECTED INTEREST GROUPS

The next consideration that the decision maker should make in developing an approach to problem solution is to identify those interest or claimant groups that will be affected by the decision. These groups should be listed and rank ordered according to priority or importance. In this way, the negative effects of a decision can be minimized because the groups affected the most will have a higher priority in the decision making process. Identification of the interest groups who will be the most directly affected is critical. If this step is carried out before the approach to problem solution is developed, the decision maker will not embark upon a course of action that will create future problems when it comes time to implement the decision.

One approach in gathering information which a decision maker might use to determine the effects of a decision on various claimant groups is to hold "public hearings." Such a hearing might entail discussions by members of a health care team on a ward, or may involve a public hearing held by a governmental agency on a proposed piece of legislation, such as national health insurance. It might also be a professional consulting with a client relative to possible decision actions. This latter case might occur when physicians or nurses discuss terminal illness with a patient to determine the patient's wishes with regard to whether or not life-saving procedures will be used to prolong life. The Living Will is an example of a claimant group, namely, the recipients of patient care, who wish to have a voice in decisions relative to death and dying, and who elect to "die with dignity," and with "no heroics."

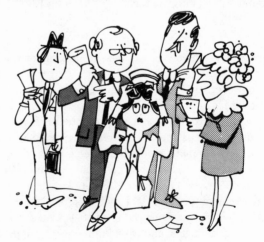

Fig. 6-4. The nurse is in a unique position to gather information from various patient care and claimant groups.

The nurse is in a unique position to gather information from various patient care and claimant groups. If nurses will gather the information carefully and use it judiciously, they will approach a problem in a more logical way and ultimately be more effective problem solvers and decision makers.

REFERENCES

1. Lewin, K.: Field theory in social science, New York, 1951, Harper & Row, Publishers.
2. Lippitt, G. L.: Organizational renewal: achieving viability in a changing world, New York, 1969, Appleton-Century-Crofts.

SUGGESTED READINGS

Moral dilemmas for practitioners in a changing society: Editorial (adapted for publication from the Annual Mary Montieth Lecture, April 17, 1972, The Annual Institute of the Loma Linda University School of Nursing Alumni Association, Loma Linda, California), J. Nurs. Admin. **3:**15-17, 1973.

Lippitt, G. L.: Overcoming people's suspicion of change, Nation's Cities (magazine of National League of Cities) **3:**15-17, 1965.

Lippitt, G. L.: Managing change: 6 ways to turn resistance into acceptance, Supervisory Management, August, 1966.

7 SPECIFYING AN APPROACH TO SOLVING THE PROBLEM

IDENTIFYING THE CONCEPTUAL FRAMEWORK FOR ATTACKING A PROBLEM

After considering constraints, capabilities, and resources, and after identifying interest groups who will be affected by a decision, the next step is to determine what approach to use in solving the problem. Basic approaches include consideration of assumptions, theories, or policies.

Three types of concern that should be considered at this point are: (1) content concerns, (2) process concerns, and (3) decision making concerns.

CONTENT CONCERNS
Assumptions

Content concerns involve assumptions that are held by individuals as they deal with problems. Assumptions that determine how a decision maker deals with problems are the product of knowledge, attitudes, values, and motivations—in short, a lifetime of cumulative psychosocial experiences. For example, certain approaches to problems of health care delivery might rest on an assumption that everyone should have health services at a reasonable cost. Another widely held assumption is that health care is a basic human right of everyone. It is important to consider the assumptions underlying any approach to problem solving if indeed the problem is to be solved. Assumptions will serve to guide the actual selection of a solution. If these assumptions remain covert, decision makers run the risk of becoming hypocritical and losing the support of those who are charged with implementing a decision.

Procedures

A second content concern deals with the procedural orientations and preferences of the decision maker or of the group that will be affected by the decisions. Problems might

---

*From Drucker, P. F.: Management: tasks, responsibilities, practices, New York, 1973, Harper & Row, Publishers.

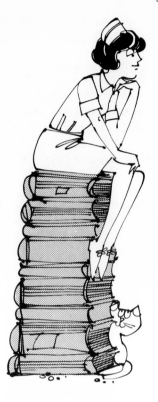

Fig. 7-1. Assumptions that determine how a decision maker deals with problems are the product of knowledge, attitudes, values, and motivations—in short, a lifetime of cumulative psychosocial experiences.

be approached through task forces, committees, teams, or nurse-client groups, or from the perspective of each individual decision maker. For example, in participatory management, a task force might be appointed to solve a problem. Another approach might be illustrated by the nurse and patient working together to resolve a patient-care problem— a client-centered approach.

Policies

The third major content concern deals with policies, regulations, and laws that will affect the decision action. This involves hospital policy, university or college policy, policies of departments, and licensing regulations as well as other types of rules that might be invoked and utilized in the problem solving process.

PROCESS CONCERNS

The second major approach category with which the decision maker is concerned is the process or the way in which he or she will actually set about solving that problem. For example, this concern involves four basic categories: (1) the organizational strategy, (2) the number of objectives considered, (3) whether or not the problem is seen as single or multi-stage, and (4) the irreversibility of the decision action.

Organizational strategy

One of the fundamental approach concerns is determining whether or not the decision maker intends to work within the existing system. Decision makers may try to reorganize the system to modify the standards so that the discrepancy between the criteria and overt actions does not occur, or they may choose to look at the level of discrepancy to see if the tolerance level needs to be reassessed.

Number of objectives considered

Decision makers need to know whether they will focus on a specific objective or set of objectives (which should be priority ranked, as we have suggested earlier). Some decision makers use a "brush fire" approach to decision objectives; that is, they rush to put out the brush fires wherever they occur, randomly focusing on objectives. This type of approach never frees the decision maker from problems because only those problems that are "burning" or drawing the most attention at a given time will be resolved.

Single or multi-stage problem

The decision maker should consider whether to solve a problem as an isolated event or consider the problem as one of a cluster or series of problems that must be solved. For example, directors of nursing service who wish to change the structure of service from a vertical, centralized structure to one which is decentralized or more horizontal may choose to deal only with the problem of structure, or they may look at a series of other problems: a beginning look at patient needs, staffing patterns to fill these needs, standards of care to determine if needs are being met, and, finally, a structure that will facilitate meeting these goals.

Irreversibility of the decision

The irreversibility of a decision will determine the type of approach that one selects. If one sees the decision as being irreversible, it is an *open-loop* decision: once the decision is made one cannot correct it by internal feedback. In an open-loop decision, more attention must be paid to the preliminary planning, pre-problem, or pre-decision making stage.

If the problem is described as *closed-loop,* the decision once made can be reversed without tremendous expenditures of resources. The decision maker at this point must determine what the potential effects of feedback might be on the decision action. The role of feedback in essence indicates whether it is going to be open-loop, that is, concerned with large policy decisions, or closed-loop, which may allow for some experimentation.

Purpose orientation of decision action

There are basically five purpose orientations to a decision action. (1) The decision can be *interim,* a brush fire type decision that puts out the flames until it is possible to return to think about the problem. (2) The decision can be *adaptive,* wherein some of the goals or procedures can be made to fit the new situation. (3) The decision can be *corrective,* that is, a problem indicates that something has gone wrong and the approach will be to make a correction and to bring the discrepancy in line with the standards. (4) The decision can be *preventive,* whereby an effort is made to prevent the occurrence of potential problems in the future. (5) The decision can be a *contingency* action, which will support other previous decisions or will provide a climate for other decisions that have been initiated.

THE DECISION MAKING CONCERNS

There are two types of decision action from which the decision maker must choose: (1) the satisficing approach, and (2) the optimizing approach.*

---

*These approaches are discussed in Chapter 3.

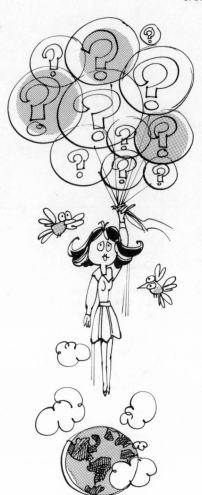

Fig. 7-2. A problem may be one of a cluster of problems.

The satisficing approach

The satisficing approach is used when a decision maker intends to select the first alternative that will solve the problem. In emergency situations this type of approach is frequently used. The expertise of the professional decision maker is usually assumed. However, it would be wasteful as a planning decision or in budget deliberations which necessitate a critical look at all possible alternatives.

The optimizing approach

An optimizing approach is one in which the decision maker looks at all possible alternatives and selects the decision that will yield the highest return for the least cost. In policy considerations, this type of approach is frequently used. Altogether the optimizing approach may take longer than a satisficing approach and may be hampered at times by a lack of appropriate information; it is the approach which should be used in approaching complex problems that affect many interest groups.

Fig. 7-3 provides a summary of the concerns the nurse manager should consider be-

Content	Assumptions	_____ _____ _____
	Procedures	Group Individual
	Policies	Hospital Licensing Labor
Process	Organizational strategy	Work within system Reorganize system Modify standards Change discrepancy levels
	Number of objectives	Specific objective Set of related objectives Random objectives
	Single or multistage	Single problem Multistage or sequence
	Irreversibility	Open-loop Closed-loop
	Purpose orientation	Interim Adaptive Corrective Preventive Contingency
Decision	Satisficing	Emergency Expediency
	Optimizing	Best for least Best available

Fig. 7-3. A checklist of approach concerns.

fore selecting an approach and before generating alternative solutions to a problem. This check sheet can be useful in helping groups discuss ideas. Objectives (ranked according to priority), constraints and capabilities, resources, and claimant groups (those groups which can be affected by a decision) should be considered at the same time.

REFERENCE

1. Drucker, P. F.: Management: tasks, responsibilities, practices, New York, 1973, Harper & Row, Publishers.

State
behavioral
objectives
and
performance
criteria

8 DEFINING DECISION OBJECTIVES AND ESTABLISHING PERFORMANCE CRITERIA

FACTORS RELATED TO DEVELOPING DECISION OBJECTIVES

Decision objectives help decision makers achieve a compromise between immediate and potential demands that are made upon them. Personal and organizational roles of the decision maker may often conflict with the direct and indirect demands of various claimant groups.

Defining decision objectives involves a consideration of three major areas: (1) the aims of the decision, (2) the interest groups or organizations who must be satisfied by a decision, and (3) the types of criteria or standards that will be used to measure the goal attainment and interest group satisfaction.

Aims of the decision

Decision makers must consider what they are striving to accomplish with their decisions. In doing so, they must consider personal goals, the goals of the various claimants or interest groups who will be affected by the decision, and the organizational aims.

Interest groups

The decision maker should be concerned with the people, interest groups, or organizations who must be satisfied with the decision. On whom will the impact of the decision fall? What priorities will be assigned to the various interests? Nurses especially need to be concerned with the impact of a decision on patients or client groups.

Establishing criteria

In establishing criteria to determine whether or not a decision objective has been met, the decision maker should consider the degrees of accomplishment. This refers to the consideration of standards and the breadth of interpretation or allowance in meeting the standards. The nature of the criteria or standards that will be used to measure goal attainment and interest group satisfaction must also be determined.

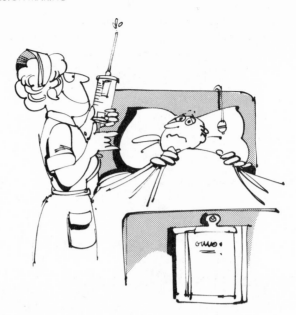

Fig. 8-1. Nurses especially need to be concerned with the impact of a decision on patients or client groups.

TWO MAJOR TYPES OF DECISION OBJECTIVES: PRESCRIPTIVE AND CONSTRAINING

Two types of decision objectives determine the nature of the criteria that are selected for measurement of goal attainment. The first type of decision objective prescribes what *should* or could be done. The other type of decision objective focuses on what *should not* be done. Some authors refer to these two types of decision goals as *prescriptive* goals and *constraining* goals.

Examples of *prescriptive decision goals* in nursing management are: (1) to increase opportunities for direct patient-centered care; (2) to improve the working environment of the unit; and (3) to develop a more effective relationship between hospital administrators and nursing service directors.

Examples of *constraining decision goals* in nursing are: (1) that nursing actions should not violate laws or nurse practice acts; and (2) that nursing care plans should not involve unnecessary risk to the patient.

Nurses need to determine whether goals are prescriptive or constraining. A set of prescriptive decision goals will necessitate congruent performance criteria, that is, performance criteria will be *positive*, directing what *can* be done to enhance achievement of the decision goal. Constraining goals focus on what *should not* be done in order to meet the decision goal. Constraining goals set the tone for performance criteria which indicate behaviors that *should not* be allowed. Typically, constraining goals specify the nature of violations of rules or regulations, or minimum standards that should be met (such as, nurse-patient ratios should not be high, or student-faculty ratios in clinical courses in a school or nursing should not rise above a certain level for safe patient care).

Decision objectives are often ambiguous. They are usually difficult to state clearly and explicitly and are often misunderstood. A common complaint is that organizations or people act in a manner that is inconsistent with stated objectives. For example, hospitals may profess high regard for quality patient care, and yet admit a larger number of patients than can be adequately cared for by a limited number of professional nursing staff. In such cases the decision maker's behavior is inconsistent with the organization's stated objectives primarily because these objectives may not be what they are proclaimed to be. In some cases the inconsistency may not be as real as it is apparent because multiple objectives are involved which necessitate compromise. Therefore no single decision goal can be fully attained without damaging the attainment of others.

DEFINING DECISION OBJECTIVES
Be specific

Establishing decision objectives is a precise procedure. Often a broad or general idea of the decision objective is stated, such as, "To make more profit." This type of a decision objective is too vague to be of use as a standard of comparison between ways of operating.

A decision objective must be precisely specified, and if possible should be located in time, place, and number. In the example given above, the decision maker should be able to state in one sentence what kind of profit, how much, when, and where. In this way the vague statement, "To make more profit," can become a more precise statement, "To make a 10% net profit after taxes in this accounting year." Such a statement gives a more precise standard that can be used as a yardstick in assessing the facts available to the manager.

Decision objectives derive from two general areas: the expected results of a decision, and the resources available in carrying out the decision. The nurse must use resources to get something done. The decision objectives that are specified are the guidelines; they will determine the use of resources in gaining advantageous results. The decision objective may be a statement of a trade-off—that is, how many resources of a certain type are needed to obtain given results.

Set priorities

Some decision objectives will be of overriding importance, while others will seem less urgent. The importance of any objective may change with time. Objectives that have been listed will influence the course of action that is selected.

Critical versus noncritical objectives. Objectives can be classified into two categories —"musts" and "wants." The critical objectives (the "musts") cannot be violated by any of the alternatives. For example, a constraining objective which limits the amount of money allocated to a given project is a critical objective in generating alternatives.

The "must" category of objectives sets maximum and minimum limits on critical resources and required results. Setting aside the "must" objectives helps the nurse to recognize and screen out impossible alternatives at the outset of the decision making process.

Noncritical objectives, those that can be classified as "wants," express relative desirability but do not set absolute limits. For example, a nurse may want to spend more time with patients than has been allocated within the work load. Nurses might like to produce higher standards of patient care than the minimum requirements set. (Striving for excellence in nursing care is a "want" objective, whereas ensuring uniformly safe care is critical.) The "want" objectives are concerned with relative advantage and disadvantage. They may involve things such as avoiding legal entanglements or continuing expenses.

If nurses can distinguish between the musts and wants of decision objectives, they can avoid the costly error of choosing an alternative action that may be later unsatisfactory because some essential ingredient was missing. If nurses can separate the critical

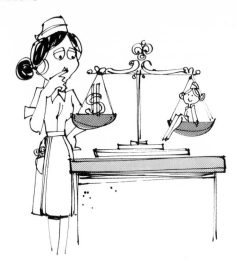

Fig. 8-2. The relative importance of each objective must be weighed.

from the noncritical objectives they will be able to look more efficiently for alternatives. The musts, or critical objectives, help to screen out poorer alternatives because any acceptable alternative must meet the standards of the critical objectives.

Weigh decision objectives

Once critical decision objectives are separated from noncritical decision objectives, the *relative importance* of each objective must be weighed. Critical objectives are considered against themselves, that is, the rank order position of each critical objective must be established in relation to each other critical objective.

A simple way to establish numerical weights for each objective is to rank order the objectives as a group going from most important to least important. To obtain a score value, merely reverse the rank order values. For example, suppose there are five critical objectives to rank:

Relative importance	Score values
First objective	5
Second objective	4
Third objective	3
Fourth objective	2
Fifth objective	1

A slightly better way to show relative importance is to start with the least critical objective and give it a weight of 1. The next step would be to ask how many times more important is the second least important objective. Using this procedure, the least important objective is taken as a standard of comparison and all the other objectives are scored against it.

Another procedure is to use a numerical scale such as a grading scale, in which a zero is failure and a 4.0 is an A or a superior score. A more discriminating scale than this is usually more desirable.

Whatever procedure is used it is critical that some assessment of relative importance is made in order to analyze the alternatives which are proposed for problem solution.

As with required objectives, the desired objectives can also be weighed according to their relative importance. Desired or noncritical objectives must not be compared to the critical objectives, which were compared among themselves. Determine the relative importance of critical objectives separately from noncritical objectives.

PROCEED FROM DECISION OBJECTIVES TO BEHAVIORAL OBJECTIVES

The next step in defining decision criteria is to determine what observable behaviors describe the decision objective. (The reader is referred to the earlier discussion of progression from goals to behavioral objectives presented in Chapter 4.) A behavioral objective narrows down the decision objective to specific behavioral terms.

Determining performance criteria

There are specific performance criteria that can be used to measure the attainment of each decision objective and subsequent behavioral objectives. Performance criteria are specific and deal with observable, measurable phenomena. There may be several performance criteria that apply to a given behavioral objective. For example, if a decision objective of a nurse is to develop a patient care plan, a subsequent behavioral objective might be to evaluate the extent to which the nurse involved the patient in developing the nursing care plan. The performance criteria established to determine whether the nurse met the stated behavioral objective might include specific questions the nurse was to ask the patient, the specific recording procedures to be used in obtaining and filing information from the patient, the number of times the nurse interacted with the patient, and the observable quality of such interactions.

Types of performance criteria

Performance criteria on which attainment of decision objectives are to be measured are basically of two types: attributes and variables. *Attributes* are characteristics that may be measured by categorical rating scales or dichotomous scaling but not by numbers. For example, yes/no and true/false rating schemes indicate categorical dichotomous attributes. Another type of categorical attribute scale might involve the categories of room temperature listed as warm, moderate, cool, and so on.

A *variable* type of performance criterion is expressed as numbers. It involves measurement on a scale of some type. An example of a variable scale is illustrated by a nine-point numerical faculty-rating scale developed by faculty to rate performance of student nurses.[1] The scale was a categorical scale on which students were rated on nineteen variables on a scale of 1-9, indicating very poor to outstanding. For example, on the variable "manual dexterity" a student who was outstanding was given a rating of 9.

Performance criteria that are capable of quantification, particularly in variable scales, are likely to be given more attention than criteria for which quantification is difficult or impossible. Quantifiable data is often easier to obtain. Variable scales also provide the decision maker latitude in the types of analysis procedures that can be used.

No measurement scheme can be completely objective. Some element of human judgment is represented in the establishment of systems of measurement. Therefore, when decision goals are translated into decision criteria complications may arise. The element of judgment in determining which criterion will describe what objective is critical. Expert opinion may vary as to which performance criterion is the best measure of a particular behavioral objective.

Measurement criteria have a profound effect on the behavior of the persons who are

DECISION OBJECTIVES	BEHAVIORAL OBJECTIVES	PERFORMANCE CRITERIA

Rank order of importance	CRITICAL (musts)	Rank	Critical	Rank	Critical
				1. _____	
		1. _____		2. _____	
				3. _____	
1. _____		2. _____		Non-CRITICAL	
				1. _____	
				2. _____	
		3. _____		3. _____	
		Non-CRITICAL		Critical	
2. _____				1. _____	
		1. _____		2. _____	
				3. _____	
		2. _____		Non-CRITICAL	
				1. _____	
				2. _____	
3. _____		3. _____		3. _____	

Non-CRITICAL (wants)	Critical	Critical
		1. _____
	1. _____	2. _____
		3. _____
1. _____	2. _____	Non-CRITICAL
		1. _____
		2. _____
	3. _____	3. _____
	Non-CRITICAL	Critical
2. _____		1. _____
	1. _____	2. _____
		3. _____
	2. _____	Non-CRITICAL
		1. _____
		2. _____
3. _____	3. _____	3. _____

Fig. 8-3. Format for developing a criterion hierarchy.

subject to the measures. Suppose, for example, that one of the objectives of a decision is to increase profitability of a hospital. Suppose a behavioral objective to be used is to lower expenditures for nursing services. A criterion might be to replace each registered nurse with a licensed vocational nurse where possible. The objective of increasing the profits of a hospital might be attained, but the overall quality of patient care might be subverted.

Establishing priorities of performance criteria

Procedures for classifying performance criteria in terms of their relative importance are the same as procedures for establishing decision objective priorities. First, separate the criteria into critical and noncritical measures. Next, establish a weighting system for the performance criteria, which can be done by rank ordering, by reverse ranking, or by scaling the critical criteria against themselves, starting with the lowest or least important of the critical criteria. The same procedure can be followed with the noncritical or desired criteria. Fig. 8-3 provides a format for listing decision objectives, behavioral objectives, and specific performance criteria.

Developing a criterion hierarchy

Decision makers may use the format for deriving a criterion hierarchy, that is, a listing of performance criteria that are subsumed under behavioral objectives and major decision objectives. A criterion hierarchy will yield a list of performance measures which the decision maker can utilize to gather information on each alternative that is proposed. Fig. 8-4 provides an example of a criterion hierarchy for selecting a job developed by a nursing student graduating from a master's degree program.*

A criterion hierarchy can be as simple or as complex as the decision maker wishes to make it. The hierarchy of performance criteria can be simply a listing of critical versus noncritical objectives and their subsequent criteria, or it can be more elaborately developed by using criterion hierarchy techniques (discussed in Chapter 10).

There are several reasons why weighting of objectives and criteria is important. First, it is beyond human capacity to evaluate performance on every decision objective simultaneously. Some objectives must be sacrificed or ignored, even if temporarily; others must take precedence.

Next, objectives that are quantifiable are likely to be given more attention than objectives for which quantification is difficult or impossible. Most people find it easier to deal with performance that is measured by numerical scaling procedures than to deal with judgments which have no numerical base.

Objectives concerned with the interests of the most powerful, articulate, or troublesome interest groups are usually given preference over objectives of less obtrusive interests. Short-term objectives are usually given priority or preference over those involving long-term commitments.

Changes in the aspirations and expectations of groups who will be affected by the decisions affect the probability of objective attainment. Since the relative importance of particular objectives changes with time, there must be a mechanism to provide for periodic reevaluation of objective priorities. When there are repetitive decisions over a long time span, this is particularly important.

---

*Fig. 8-4 is derived from Mary S. Meister's project report for Dr. K. Claus' course on managerial decision making (Psychology 205), University of California, San Francisco, Spring, 1974.

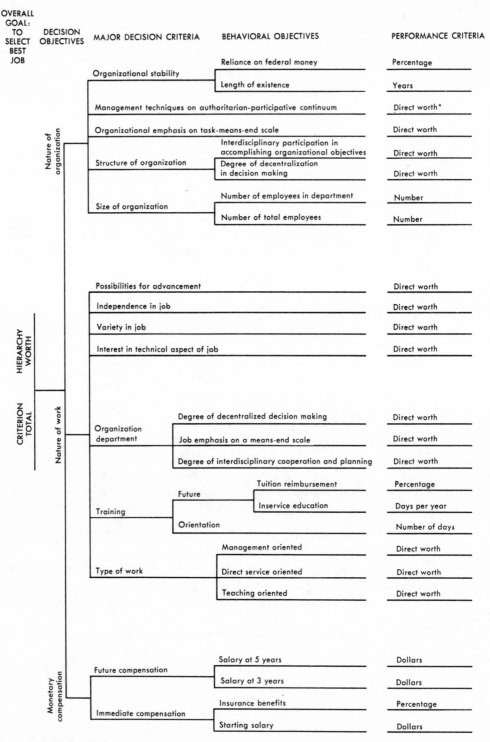

Fig. 8-4. Criterion hierarchy used by a graduate nursing student to select a place of employment.

*Direct worth refers to a direct percent type, numerical estimate of the subjective (personally perceived) worth of a given criterion to the decision maker.

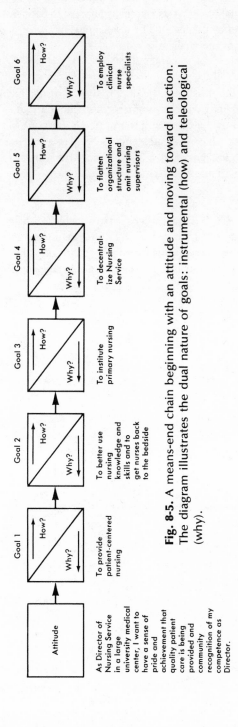

Fig. 8-5. A means-end chain beginning with an attitude and moving toward an action. The diagram illustrates the dual nature of goals: instrumental (how) and teleological (why).

RECONCILING CONTRADICTORY GOALS

Each goal has two aspects: an instrumental aspect and a teleological aspect. The instrumental or "how" aspect looks forward to behavior and seeks to determine how the purpose is to be achieved. The teleological or "why" looks back and seeks to determine the purpose of the goals.

The means-end chain

Fig. 8-5 illustrates the dual nature of goals. The means-end chain starts from an attitude and ends with a specific recommendation for action. Moving from the attitude to the first goal in the chain and then to higher order goals, it becomes apparent that there is a sequence which indicates how the various goals are to be obtained. The sequence begins with the last goal and moves toward the attitudes. This type of a procedure is used by many in an attempt to find answers to "why" questions.

The means-end tree

Fig. 8-5 illustrates a goal chain called a means-end chain, which is a linear series without any branches. Usually there are alternative means for achieving the ends. Alternative means can be displayed in a means-ends hierarchy which resembles a tree or pyramid. Fig. 8-6 illustrates how a single higher level objective gives rise to multiple lower level goals.

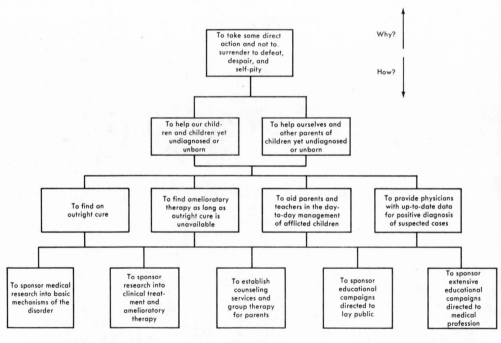

Fig. 8-6. A means-end hierarchy. Four levels of a pyramid means-end associated with the objectives of the founders of a medical research foundation organized to support research and education leading to greater knowledge of a rare, often fatal, inborn metabolic disorder of children. (Adapted from Easton, A.: Complex managerial decision making involving multiple objectives, New York, 1973, John Wiley & Sons, Inc.)

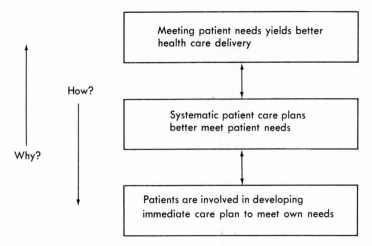

Fig. 8-7. A means-end chain can help to reconcile seemingly contradictory goals.

Resolving disputes or confusion

A means-end tree is helpful in resolving disputes or in clarifying confusion about decision objectives. Nurses frequently differ in decision objectives relative to patient care. For example, one nurse may feel that meeting patient needs is the most important goal and that the nurse professional is in the best position to make judgments about patient care plans. Another nurse may argue that enabling the patient to be a primary decision maker in his own immediate care should be paramount. These two objectives may not be mutually exclusive, but can be related to each other by a means-end chain. See Fig. 8-7 for an illustration of how these two seemingly disparate goals can be related to each other by a means-end chain. Very often seemingly contradictory goals can be reconciled by recognizing their place on a means-end goal chain or within a means-end hierarchy.

Decision makers can make identification of complex decision objectives easier if they construct a means-end chain or hierarchy for each major objective or overall objective. Some objectives will fit in an upper level, while others will fit at middle or lower levels of a chain. Overlap will occur because some means will simultaneously satisfy more than one end.

REFERENCES

1. Bailey, J. T., McDonald, F., and Claus, K. E.: An experiment in nursing curriculums at a university, Belmont, Calif., 1972, Wadsworth Publishing Co.
2. Easton, A.: Complex managerial decision making involving multiple objectives, New York, 1973, John Wiley & Sons, Inc.

SUGGESTED READING

Vargas, J. S.: Writing worthwhile behavioral objectives, New York, 1972, Harper & Row, Publishers.

Man owes his success to his creativity.

DE BONO*

9 GENERATING ALTERNATIVE SOLUTIONS

Previous chapters have described a number of problem solving procedures and steps. The steps presented are indeed requisite to systematically approaching problems, but additional steps are needed for effective problem solution. As we have noted, a satisficing solution is acceptable in some situations that require immediate action; however, many problem situations in the delivery of care require a more complex and time-consuming approach. These situations may require a creative approach—new ideas about solutions to the problem.

SOURCES OF ALTERNATIVES

Careful planning and thorough search for alternative solutions to problems is a critical process in putting together original, effective solutions and in bringing about change in the delivery of care. In a search for alternative solutions to a problem, there are a number of resources available which should be considered: (1) past experience; (2) experience of colleagues; (3) the opinions of groups who will be affected by the final decision; (4) suggestions generated by special groups and/or task forces who are organized for problem solving; and (5) consultation from experts outside the organization or perhaps outside the nursing profession.

TECHNIQUES FOR BUILDING A CREATIVE CLIMATE

The next step in developing creative solutions is to provide a climate in which participants feel free to contribute new and unusual ideas. Creative is a key word describing the quality of a solution that will satisfy the critical criteria. A creative solution is one that is both unique and valuable. The uniqueness and value may be to the individual, the group, the organization, or society. Creativity can be encouraged or discouraged by the climate maintained in the problem solving process.

---

*From de Bono, E.: Lateral thinking for management, London, 1971, American Management Association, p. 1.

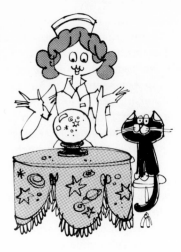

Fig. 9-1. In a search for alternative solutions to a problem, there are a number of resources available.

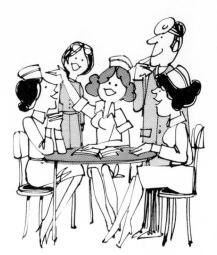

Fig. 9-2. In brainstorming, ideas stimulate other ideas.

Collective creativity: brainstorming

The concept of brainstorming (using more than one brain to "storm" an idea) comes from the business world, but has almost universal application. The main assumption underlying the technique is that ideas stimulate other ideas: one person may have a good suggestion, which another person hears, and he in turn thinks of an effective idea. The second idea might have never occurred without the stimulation of the first idea.

Maximizing effectiveness. A small number of participants in a brainstorming group has been found to be the most effective (between five and ten members). If a larger group is used, cooperation tends to deteriorate. Brainstorming is a particularly effective procedure to use when a problem has been narrowly defined. Another advantage of brainstorming sessions is that a large number of solutions can be generated which may produce one or two outstanding alternatives.

Experience has shown that results from brainstorming sessions depend on what is sometimes referred to as a "hard specification of a problem." A brainstorming group must have the problem clearly defined in order to be productive. Labels such as "staffing problems" or "problems of student dissatisfaction" will lead groups astray and produce feelings of frustration.

Groups should also be instructed to address themselves to only *one problem*. More than one problem in a session can prove to be a disaster. Lack of focus produces confusion and conflict, leading to frustration of group members who have spent unproductive time.

Leadership. The first task in planning a brainstorming session is to select a leader and participants. The quality of the results of brainstorming sessions depends largely on the effectiveness of the leader. Without effective leadership to monitor the process, the most capable and creative members of the group may be unable to function.

Participants. Participants from all levels of nursing service or the health care delivery system should be included in a brainstorming session. Frequently, it is helpful to include one or more persons from outside the nursing profession—a social worker, psychologist, sociologist, volunteer, consumer—whose orientation to the problem might be somewhat different from that of nurses.

Atmosphere and setting. One of the primary tasks of the leader is to keep the session informal and lively. There are a number of ways to do this. One way to create a relaxed atmosphere is to schedule a midmorning meeting with coffee and a "snack" or to plan a luncheon meeting. The feeling of informality is critical because participants need to be confident that what they may say will not be taken with undue seriousness.

The primary focus of a brainstorming session is to assist the members of the group to produce as many ideas as possible. Ten ideas, however bizarre, are preferred to one thoughtfully considered, comprehensive suggestion. The leader plays the role of a referee whose function is to "keep the ball in play." Participants are encouraged to disperse with formality, to let ideas "fly," to relax and "free float."

Ground rules. One of the most important ground rules in a brainstorming session is: Do not pass judgment on the ideas presented. The purpose of the group effort is to create, not to criticize. Ideas that may seem silly are actually important and have their place —they have a real function in keeping the session relaxed, in dispelling tension. Members who insist on criticizing ideas proposed (possibly as a substitute for offering suggestions of their own) need to be dealt with firmly and reminded of the ground rules.

Evaluation may creep in under various disguises: "We've already said that"; "That probably costs too much"; "Nobody would go along with that"; "That's been tried before and it didn't work"; "That's a dumb idea." These are comments that have a negative effect. They make group members evaluate their own ideas before they blurt them out, which means that many ideas go unexpressed. The leader should not only squelch criticism, but should encourage zaniness in ideas. Developing a mood for brainstorming and generating zany ideas may be difficult for some members, especially at first. The urge to evaluate may be all but irresistible to some individuals, while others may find generating zany ideas, particularly in an institutional setting, somewhat ludicrous.

Function of recorder. To ensure that results of brainstorming are not lost, one person should act as record keeper, with instructions to note every idea that is generated. Assigning a recorder has been found preferable to the use of a tape recorder, which tends to intimidate and inhibit some members. After the session, participants may wish to have a list of the ideas that were generated; such a list should be provided.

Results. With the guidance of an effective leader, brainstorming sessions are known to work extremely well. Not only are potentially useful ideas generated, but participants tend to be enthusiastic and to feel rewarded about their experience. The informal, non-judgmental atmosphere generates a feeling of importance among all levels of management represented in the group.

Two factors that are believed to contribute to the success of brainstorming sessions are the absence of criticism and the contagion that results from ideas being allowed to influence each other. Some of the most outstanding ideas from these sessions are combinations of ideas generated by several people, put together by another person, and modified by still another. Ideas can indeed be multiplied by the brainstorming process and creative alternatives to problems generated through such a participative endeavor.

Guided group creativity: synectics

While brainstorming depends on the creativity of participants helping each other to spark ideas, an approach called synectics (the joining together of unrelated elements) gives structured directions on how to produce those ideas.

Assumptions. In theory, synectics maintains that: (1) if people understand the psychological processes which are involved in the creative process, they can enhance their own creative efficiency; (2) the emotional side of the creative process is more significant than the intellectual; (3) the irrational element is more important then the rational; and, (4) when emotional, irrational components are understood (as they can be), the chances for successful problem solving will be enhanced.

Training. When groups are trained in synectics, they undergo formalized phases of progress. Nurses may not want to expend the energy or resources for this formalized training, but they may abstract principles which can be applied to finding alternative solutions. When a group is trained in synectics, progress is evaluated by analyzing the problem solutions that have been proposed. Solutions to technical problems are particularly amenable to synectics procedures. Perhaps this is because these solutions can be assessed more objectively than can certain other types of poblem solutions, such as those proposed for long-range policy decisions.[4] Nevertheless, the steps followed lend themselves to wide application. Groups who use synectics techniques usually include people from various backgrounds to ensure a variety of perceptions of the problem.

Ground rules. In synectics, it is helpful to forget that the problem is "old hat" and that one has encountered the problem many times. A conscious effort is required to make that which is familiar seem strange, or to look at a situation with fresh eyes like the eyes of a child. In the practice of synectics, four different but related procedures or mechanisms have been recognized which facilitate a new look at an old problem. These have been identified as characteristic of what happens when creative ideas are found.

Procedures. Creativity is a dynamic, moving process and not a static fact which can be understood by examining the end result. By studying the kinds of thoughts that creative individuals have reported as leading to their insights, certain modes of thought emerge which seem to be part of the psychological processes of creativity. These include: (1) personal analogy; (2) direct analogy; (3) symbolic analogy; and (4) fantasy analogy. From the perspective of synectics, these four types of analogy are prerequisites to problem solving.

The assumption underlying the use of these procedures is that they can be consciously followed and that they can initiate or spark the creative process. People who think of creativity as a special gift that someone either has or does not have from the moment of birth may resist this somewhat mechanistic view of creativity. Within the framework of synectics, however, these procedures can help a group generate creative solutions. With practice, synectics will become a way of perceiving personal problems and health care problems, and perhaps contribute to new perceptions of man's environment.

Personal analogy. When individuals are able to temporarily forget the elements of a problem and become a part of the problem, they are using personal analogy. This is one way to make a familiar problem appear strange. Scientists have used this approach with marked success. The scientist who was able to discover the structure of benzene did not

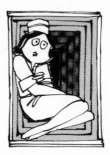

Fig. 9-3. Personal analogy involves becoming a part of the problem.

find the answer by thinking about molecules but by analogy to other things—what it "felt like" to *be* inside the benzene molecule. In reporting what they have seen, children often use this technique—the small boy talking about the space flight films he has seen becomes the rocket himself. Try telling another person how to tie a particular knot. If you do not have a piece of string to demonstrate the technique you may soon find your fingers becoming part of the knot, again by personal analogy.

Direct analogy. When data or observed facts are compared unchanged from one situation to another, the mechanism of direct analogy is used. Many times nature provides models for technology. A saw may have originated as a direct analogy to teeth. Human and animal teeth break if they are used on extremely hard substances, but a saw made of a harder substance has certain advantages over teeth. A button hook, used when everyone wore shoes with tiny buttons and loops to be fastened, was probably conceived of by direct analogy to a bent finger. A human finger was too large to fit conveniently around the tiny loops, but a hook with a very small bend in it could be used with ease.

Symbolic analogy. Symbolic analogy is different from both personal and direct analogy, which are both descriptive. In some ways, symbolic analogy is similar to a gestalt response: patterns and similarities emerge between things that once appeared unrelated.

Nurses may not be as familiar with the metaphors of poetry as are specialists in the humanities. But there is no reason that nurses cannot become comfortable with the poetic way of thinking or with practice acquire facility in seeing things in a new, symbolic relation to other things. Symbolic analogy may be a source of understanding patient care problems. The patient with undiagnosable chest pains may indeed be suffering from a "broken heart." Unexplainable dermatological problems of patients may be a manifestation of a patient who "has something under his skin."

Fantasy analogy. Since the pioneering work of Freud, psychologists have recognized a relationship between creative thought and the fulfillment of wishes. According to Freud, part of what the artist does is to express the satisfaction of a wish. A competent artist can find satisfaction in his work because in a fanciful, fantastic way it satisfies an original wish.

Fantasy analogy has been used successfully in the resolution of technical problems in science. To launch into a fantasy analogy approach, the problem at hand must be considered. Next the following question should be raised: "In my most bizarre imaginings, how would I want this solution to work?" As with the other mechanisms of synectics, this approach is directed at stimulating the creative processes.

Lateral thinking

A mother had five children and eleven apples. How did she divide the apples evenly among the children?*

---

*Answer: she made applesauce.

This children's riddle illustrates lateral thinking. Individual and group problem solving efforts are often characterized by certain assumptions which one holds relative to thought processes, and which have been described as vertical thinking. The concept of vertical thinking describes the logical progression from step 1 to step 2—the necessity for each step in a logical progression to be correct if subsequent steps are to be valid, or the reliance on "yes/no" answers to questions. Vertical thinking appears to be logical—the right way to solve problems.

What is lateral thinking? Edward de Bono, a medical doctor and psychologist, criticized vertical thinking.[2,3] He suggested that a new type of thinking is needed for creative solutions to problems, which he referred to as lateral thinking. The concept of lateral thinking is presented as a deliberate jump away from the logical progression of moving from step 1 to step 2. de Bono maintained that there are situations in which the traditional approach of vertical thinking cannot produce satisfactory solutions. Lateral thinking may involve standing the problem "on its head" or "turning the problem inside out." This is similar to the synectics concept of making the familiar seem strange.

How does it work? Guidelines for using concepts of lateral thinking include the following:

1. Try to think of other ways in which the problem can be stated.
2. In a relaxed frame of mind, recall the "far out" ideas that come to mind as solutions.
3. Try to invert the problem.
4. Think up another problem that could take the place of the current one.
5. Change the place of the emphasis from one part of the problem to another.

These steps may not be easy to follow at first. There may be a certain amount of inertia and of comfortable familiarity in using the old patterns of vertical thinking; however, they must be temporarily suspended if lateral thinking is to be used.

The terminology of lateral thinking may be new, but the phenomenon has been intuitively understood for a long time. A form of lateral thinking is depicted in a story associated with Samuel Clemens. As a young man, Clemens wanted very much to be a riverboat pilot on the Mississippi. when he approached a captain about being hired he was asked, "Do you know where the snags are in this stretch of the river?" "Nope," answered Clemens, "but I know where they ain't." He got the job.*

Usefulness. Lateral thinking is potentially useful to both individuals and groups in generating alternatives to problem solution. there are similarities and differences between lateral thinking and brainstorming. Lateral thinking is similar to brainstorming in its encouragement of offbeat ideas, but different in its reluctance to accept the proposed definition of the problem.

DIFFERENCES BETWEEN INDIVIDUAL AND GROUP PROBLEM SOLVING

Techniques introduced in this chapter—brainstroming, synectics, and lateral thinking—are important and useful but not always interchangeable. Some approaches may be well suited to individual problem solving, others to group effort. The nature of a particular problem situation, the personalities of the people involved, and the characteristics of the leader should be considered in choosing an approach.

---

* See Chapter 5 for discussion of the importance of determining "what the problem is not" in problem definition.

Individuals

Basically, the search for alternatives in problem solution can be outlined in the following steps when the search is being conducted and approached by an individual: (1) use of a basic strategy; (2) recollection of information that is relevant, and manipulation (recombining in new ways) of information; and (3) exploring information in terms of the hypotheses involved in the goal of problem solution.

Groups

When a group is solving a problem, attention shifts to different steps: (1) having discussions to seek and develop alternatives; (2) use of summarizing discussions (this may be sparked by a naive question such as "I'm not sure I've followed everything to this point; can somebody straighten me out?"); (3) reconciliation of suggestions that oppose each other.*

In comparing group with individual attempts at finding creative alternative solutions, it is difficult to say which approach is more effective. There appears to be no clear consensus among experts. Some argue that groups are more efficient at searches because they can eliminate erroneous ideas quickly; however, research findings do not support this theory.

Some of the assumptions underlying group participation in decision making are currently being analyzed and questioned. One investigation reported that it does not necessarily follow that involvement in decision making will encourage an individual to experience greater commitment to the organization.[1] Further, it was found that some individuals are required to participate in too many decisions and consequently feel overloaded and ineffective in the decision making process.

The "decision load" of nurses and health professionals is indeed unusually heavy. One way of making the "decision load" lighter is to provide the problem solver with a systematic way of defining and solving problems. Another way is to make nurse managers aware of a tendency to overload certain individuals with more decisions than they can effectively attend to, which results in ineffective decision making.

---

*The means-end chain discussed in Chapter 8 is a useful procedure here.

REFERENCES

1. Alutto, J. A., and Belasco, J. A.: A typology for participation in organizational decision making, Administrative Science Quarterly **17:**117-125, 1972.
2. de Bono, E.: Lateral thinking for management, London, 1971, American Management Association.
3. de Bono, E.: Po: a device for successful thinking, New York, 1972, Simon & Schuster.
4. Gordon, W. J.: Synectics: the development of creative capacity, New York, 1961, Collier.

SUGGESTED READINGS

Anderson, H. H., editor: Creativity and its cultivation, New York, 1959, Harper & Row, Publishers.

Osborne, A. F.: Your creative power, New York, 1948, Charles Scribner & Son.

Osborne, A. F.: Applied imagination, New York, 1963, Charles Scribner & Son.

Parnes, S. J.: Creative behavior guidebook, New York, 1967, Charles Scribner & Son.

Taylor, C. W., editor: Climate for creativity, New York, 1972, Pergamon Press.

The understanding that underlies the right decision grows out of the clash and conflict of divergent opinions and out of the serious consideration of competing alternatives.

P. L. DRUCKER*

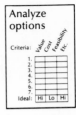

10 ANALYZING DECISION ALTERNATIVES

After completing the first six steps presented in the Claus-Bailey Systems Model, the next step is to determine what program of action, when adopted and implemented, will correct the discrepancy or problem. As discussed in Chapter 7, the decision maker can opt to search for only one acceptable solution (the satisficing approach) or to search for a number of solutions from which to choose the best solution (the optimizing approach).

THE NECESSITY FOR ANALYSIS OF ALTERNATIVES

The first alternative which comes to mind may not be the best. In most cases the decision maker can think of several ways of dealing with the problem. Each alternative may have both strong and weak points, or may favor one interest group and disfavor others. To avoid this dilemma, it is necessary to evaluate all alternative solutions on each of the relevant criteria.

In the section that follows, two basic approaches to the analysis of decision alternatives will be presented. The first approach is relatively simple and requires very little time. The other procedure is time-consuming and should be used for evaluating complex situations when long-range and large-scale decisions are to be made. The techniques described in the latter procedure apply to situations in which the decision maker wishes to utilize the input of a group or seeks the input from a number of experts or consultants.

PREPARING DATA FOR ANALYSIS OF ALTERNATIVES
The matrix form

To facilitate analysis of proposed alternatives, it is necessary to test data and to place available data in a format that lends itself to comparison. An effective way to do this is to cast the data into a matrix form, illustrated in Fig. 10-2. † As noted in the illustration, the alternatives are listed in a column on the left-hand side. Associated with each alternative is a score or category rating which expresses how that alternative is evaluated on each criterion measure. The criteria are listed across the top of the page, with the critical

---

*From Drucker, P. L.: Management: tasks, responsibilities, practices, New York, 1973, Harper & Row, Publishers, p. 471.

† See also cases presented in Part two of this book.

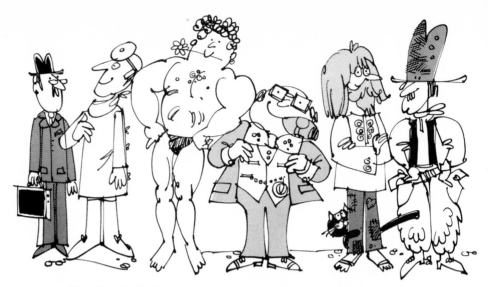

Fig. 10-1. Each alternative may have both strong and weak points.

Decision performance criteria

Alternatives	Critical			Noncritical		Scores
	Cost	Feasibility	Risk	Comfort	Attractiveness	
1._____						
2._____						
3._____						
4._____						
5._____						
Ideal	Low	High	Low	Mod-high	Mod-high	

Fig. 10-2. Example of an outcome matrix.

criteria listed first. The score assigned to each alternative on each criterion measure may be in numerical form or expressed as a general evaluation such as "High," "Medium," or "Low." To aid comparison with the desired outcome or decision objective, the bottom line can be used to indicate the values which are ideal or which the decision maker wishes to approximate.

Determining the best alternative. When using the procedure outlined above, the next step is to circle those score values in the matrix which correspond with the ideal or desired outcome listed on the bottom of the table.

Add up the number of circled scores and indicate the total in the specified column. Inspection of total scores will enable the decision maker to quickly decide which alterna-

Decision performance criteria

Alternative	Critical			Noncritical		Scores
	Cost to player	Knowledge needed to play	Risk	Psychologi-cal comfort of player	Attractive-ness	
Tiddly winks	(Low)	(Low)	(Low)	(High)	Low	4
Poker	High	Mod	High	Low	(High)	1
Scrabble	(Low)	Mod	(Low)	(Mod)	(Mod)	4
Canasta	Mod	Mod	Mod	(Mod)	(Mod)	2
Monopoly	(Low)	(Low)	Mod	(Mod)	(High)	4
Ideal	Low	Low	Low	Mod-high	Mod-high	

Fig. 10-3. Example showing how an outcome matrix is used to evaluate alternatives (to select a party game).

tive most closely meets the ideal in solving the problem. Fig. 10-3 illustrates how this procedure is used.

Although the above procedure can be done relatively easily, it is not the end of the process. Suppose decision makers are faced with a tied score or with a situation in which they intuitively feel that one alternative is preferable even though it does not show the highest total points. At this point it is necessary to apply *decision rules*. Although decision rules will be discussed in the next chapter, we feel it necessary to inform the reader that the decision rules which form the basis for the decision action taken stem from the approach which the problem solver specified in step 4 and which was discussed in Chapter 7.*

Merit ordering systems

The second major procedure for analyzing proposed alternatives is considerably more time-consuming and complex. A more complex procedure is necessary when the decision maker must take responsibility for long-range decisions or decisions which involve considerable expenditure of resources and which will affect the interests of many people.

The basic approach in this type of decision analysis is to develop *merit ordering* systems for the various alternatives presented. Merit ordering implies the combination of various evaluation rules and involves the estimation of an outcome for a given alternative on a given criterion.

Worth assessment. The estimation or assessment of worth must also be considered.

---

*For example, a pediatric nurse specialist concerned with teaching a child how to use a kidney dialysis machine makes a different set of decisions if learning is perceived as a gestalt-type cognitive process than if learning is perceived as a stimulus-response process. In the first instance the nurse selects alternatives which produce a presentation telling the child all about the machine, how it is used, why it is used, etc. The second approach produces a programmed presentation composed of a series of activities or questions wherein the child learns by increments.

Alternatives	Critical		Noncritical	Scores
1. _____	probability / value	probability / value	probability / value	
2. _____	probability / value	probability / value	probability / value	
3. _____	probability / value	probability / value	probability / value	
Ideal				

Fig. 10-4. Example of a payoff matrix.

Synonyms for assessed worth are desirability, attractiveness, or positive value. In decision theory the concept of worth is known as *utility*. Utility may be either positive or negative. *Positive utility* has the capability of either directly or indirectly satisfying human needs that contribute to the attainment of individual, group, or organizational goals. *Negative utility* (called disutility in decision theory) frustrates need satisfaction or goal attainment and reduces the feeling of well-being.

Estimates of outcome also involve assumptions about certainty, risk, and uncertainty. By assigning a number to the expected outcome of various decision alternatives on various criteria, the decision maker can provide an underlying estimate of the certainty and risk involved in attaining the expected outcome.

The payoff matrix. The table used for testing the data in complex decision analysis is called a *payoff matrix** (Fig. 10-4). Although the payoff matrix is somewhat similar in construction to the simple matrix described above, the payoff matrix is constructed with cells in which the decision maker places two numbers: one to indicate the probability of the given outcome, and the other to indicate the value of that outcome according to some system for estimating worth.

Utility estimation. Two types of reporting scores can be placed in payoff matrix. One is an actual *numerical value*, which can be obtained directly from the criteria for each alternative (for example, dollars, numbers of months required, or distance).

The second type of utility estimation is called a *direct worth estimate*, which is made on a quality basis. The decision maker assigns a number to the score on given criteria

---

*A payoff matrix can be constructed from a criteron hierarchy. See Chapter 8.

attained by a particular alternative. Examples of this type of quality score would be a variable such as climate, or degree of person's involvement, or the type of nursing school that a student may have attended. A numerical score cannot be attained on a quality-type variable. These variables are also called attributes or categorical variables. A relative number must be generated which describes how a particular alternative scores on that type of variable. These are subjective score values and will vary in the judgment of different individuals.

PROCEDURES FOR SCORING ALTERNATIVES ON THE CRITERIA

When analyzing complex alternatives involving multiple objectives it is helpful to utilize all of the available professional input. The decision maker can do this by holding meetings or by asking for opinions from various persons whose input is desired. The decision maker should also include in the analysis of alternatives those people who will be charged with implementing a decision. The following section describes some procedures for utilizing input from many sources when analyzing proposed alternative solutions to a problem.

Creation of utility functions

Estimating worth. A utility function is a curve which describes how a group feels about the value of a given alternative. To create a utility function, the following procedure is useful:

1. Each person involved in the estimation provides an opinion of what the admissible score range should be. Suppose a health care team is considering the purchase of a respirator. In terms of dollar cost, one group member may see as acceptable the range from $10,000 to $50,000, with everything above and below these limits being unacceptable. Perhaps another person in the group feels that $8,000 to $40,000 would be sufficient limits. After obtaining several estimates of the adequate range, the group leader averages the scores and determines the score values upon which the group members can agree.

2. The agreed-upon values are then plotted on a graph; the curve represented by the plot points is called the utility function. The utility function for the above example is shown in Fig. 10-5.

Relative criterion weights

A systematic method for scoring alternatives that have been generated provides the decision maker with a rationale for defending the decision. The defense rests on the notion that the criteria and weighting systems were developed by group consensus.

The acceptable relative weight of each criterion against the other criteria can be determined by assigning a percentage weight to each criterion. Weights for each criterion category (each set of branches on a criterion hierarchy) must add up to 1.0 (or 100%).

Another procedure for developing relative weights for the various performance criteria is to rank order the criteria. Table 1 indicates the procedure for this approach. Note that reverse rank scores were given the various criteria. In other words, the highest ranking criterion obtained the highest score.

Composite relative weights. Suppose the decision maker wants to adjust the relative weights by a rank order weighting system, in order to incorporate two types of evaluation procedures. For example, in an examination perhaps an educator wishes to give the student credit for effort in terms of the amount of energy spent on discussing given questions in an examination, while at the same time allow for rating of the process repre-

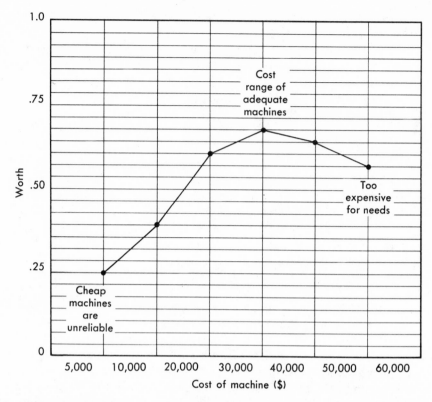

Fig. 10-5. Utility function for estimated worth scores for purchasing a respirator.

Table 1. A rank order procedure for developing relative criterion weights

Performance criteria	Rank order	Reverse rank order
Cost	1	5
Feasibility	2	4
Risk	3	3
Comfort	4	2
Attractiveness	5	1

sented by the questions according to importance in professional practice. In this case a relative or percentage weight would be used to determine the traditional grading of an examination—the number of references used and the like—whereas each question could be rank ordered with regard to its importance to professional practice.

Alternative scores

The procedure for computing a score for a given alternative on a set of criteria is shown in Table 2. The relative weights of each criterion (that is, the relative importance of each criterion compared to the other criteria) is multiplied by the utility score that the given alternative earns on each criterion. The utility score, as you may remember, was obtained

Table 2. Procedure for developing score values for complex alternatives

Performance criteria	Relative weight*	×	Utility score†	=	Score on criteria
Cost	5	×	_____	=	_____
Feasibility	4	×	_____	=	_____
Risk	3	×	_____	=	_____
Comfort	2	×	_____	=	_____
Attractiveness	1	×	_____	=	_____

*Relative weight refers to the relative importance of each criterion compared to all the other criteria.
†Utility refers to the subjective value of an alternative. This is the value of that alternative compared to any other possible alternative that the decision maker might consider. For example, in salary range a salary of $10,000 might be valued one half as highly as a salary of $20,000; $5,000 might not even be within the admissible range, therefore rating a 0.

from a plot of the ideas regarding the value range of the criterion. These ideas or estimates either can be the product of individual thought or can be determined by group consensus.

Total criterion scores. The total weighted score for the alternative on that set of criteria is obtained by adding up all of the products of the relative weights and criterion scores (last column in Table 2). Depending upon the decision rule which has been established (to be discussed later), the total will be found acceptable or not acceptable.

Figures of merit. A figure of merit is an index number that is representative of the relative merit, worth, attractiveness, or desirability of the given alternatives. A figure of merit (FOM) can be calculated for each alternative presented. This is done by multiplying the relative weights by adjusting factors (such as a reverse rank score). The composite weighting system described above is a procedure for developing figures of merit (FOM's).[2, 4]

The alternative having the highest figure of merit will be the alternative selected unless decision rules indicate another procedure. For example, in grading examinations there may be a cutoff point above which figures of merit are acceptable and below which they are unacceptable or failures.

USING THE COMPUTER TO AID IN MAKING COMPLEX MANAGERIAL DECISIONS

When large criterion hierarchies and complicated weighting systems are involved, it may be difficult to compute all the necessary figures in order to make a decision. In such cases the computer can be an aid in expediting the procedure of decision analysis. This is particularly true in hospital admissions, graduate school admissions, or other cases in which a procedure, once established, can be reapplied in many cases. These procedures can also be utilized in monitoring various physiological processes. Nurses may become involved in helping to develop some of the weighting systems used in making particular types of patient care decisions based upon these analysis procedures.

PROCEDURES WHICH USE A DECISION ANALYSIS APPROACH IN SOLVING HEALTH CARE DELIVERY PROBLEMS

There are two basic procedures that are utilized by hospital administrators to analyze various aspects of health care delivery. Each of these systems incorporates elements of the problem solving process and decision analysis sequence, which have already been discussed. One of these procedures is cost benefit analysis, the other is cost effectiveness analysis.

Cost benefit analysis (CBA)

Cost benefit analysis is used to assess the worth of projects when it is important to consider repercussions that may occur in the future. Cost benefit analysis involves essentially two stages: (1) the enumeration and evaluation of all the costs and benefits expected from a project; and (2) a comparison of costs and benefits. Since costs and benefits will normally be in different forms, the analyst makes them commensurate by reducing them to common monetary values.

This form of analysis relies heavily on quantification of costs and benefits, and loses its power when important costs and benefits cannot be expressed in monetary terms. Usually these unquantifiable factors are omitted from the computations and are accounted for by narrative, which has limitations. A common practice is to prepare balance sheets showing costs and benefits for all the identifiable interests that can be quantified. Cost benefit studies can be used to pinpoint potential trouble spots if one group receives the benefits and another group pays the costs. When such real and perceived inequities are discovered, the project sponsors can expect difficulties unless equalization can be achieved by some other means.

There are effects that cannot be compensated by money or another satisfactory equivalent. Loss of life is such a noncompensable situation. Ordinary monetary equivalents cannot adequately reflect the frustration or disutilities with such noncompensable effects. Yet these effects cannot be quantified and there is danger that they will be given insufficient weight in the formation of the cost benefit ratio or cost benefit balance.

Health service delivery systems have utilized cost benefit analysis extensively.[3] There are, however, complications and subtleties involved in cost benefit analysis, such as predicting possible effects or dealing with pressure groups who may attempt to influence the analysis.

Cost effectiveness analysis (CEA)

Another type of analysis that uses systematic techniques is called cost effectiveness analysis. In this procedure the alternatives for achieving specified objectives are compared. The purpose of the analysis is to find the alternative that will attain the objective at the least amount of financial expenditure. For example, a hospital administrator or architect may seek to find the most economical ward arrangement of patients in order to provide services for a given quantity of patients at a given quality level. In cost effectiveness analysis, the cost is also expressed in dollars. Often the end result is a ratio of units of performance per dollar of outlay.

Both of the above procedures evaluate alternatives on many criteria that have been made equivalent (usually by reducing to monetary terms). The procedure we discussed earlier also employs a procedure for arriving at figures of merit (FOM) for each alternative evaluated by the criteria listed. In this way many types of criteria can be compared. Many complex decisions have at least one cost objective but often have many other types of objectives which are not so easily quantifiable and must be based on estimates, derived by the decision maker either from consensus of a group or by personal expertise.[2, 5]

REFERENCES

1. Drucker, P. L.: Management: tasks, responsibilities, practices, New York, 1973, Harper & Row, Publishers.
2. Easton, A.: Complex managerial decisions involving multiple objectives, New York, 1970, John Wiley & Sons, Inc.
3. Klarman, H. E.: The economics of health, New York, 1965, Columbia University Press.
4. Miller, J. R. III: Professional decision making: a procedure for evaluating complex alternatives, New York, 1970, Praeger.
5. Packer, H. A.: Applying cost-effectiveness concepts to the community health system, Journal of Operations Research Society of America **16:**227-253, 1968.

Choose:
apply
decision
rules
A. _____
B. _____
C. _____
D. _____

11 MAKING A CHOICE

Approaches to problem solutions were discussed in Chapter 7. Steps involved in selecting an approach consisted of analyzing constraints and capabilities, generating hypotheses as to the cause of the problem, and formulating decision rules (based on assumptions about nursing, life, learning, and so on) to use in selecting a course of action.

If decision makers carefully consider the approach to decision making prior to determining decision objectives and criteria, decision rules may already be built into the process. If assumptions, purposes, or goals are built into the weighting of the decision criteria then the alternative with the highest score (be it a figure of merit, rank, mean score, or other indicator) should be the best alternative to solve the problem. This is the reason it is important to articulate all underlying assumptions when discussing the approach. Some of these assumptions and orientations may be the very factors that determine how a person will make a decision.

APPLYING DECISION RULES

A decision rule is used to select an alternative on the basis of given purposes, goals, or assumptions. Lee defines a decision rule or decision principle as "a rule for specifying which of the set of possible decision is rational (or optimal)."[2] Whether or not a decision is judged to be rational depends upon the decision rule or principle employed by the decision maker.

Function of decision rules

Failure to specify decision rules often accounts for those situations in which a person who, after going through a complicated analysis of alternatives, still experiences an intuitive preference for an alternative which simply does not rank as high as another alternative. Although there may be a miscalculation somewhere, this type of situation could point to the fact that all of the underlying assumptions and objectives were not examined earlier.

The time-consuming job of redeveloping decision criteria may be difficult or impos-

---

[*]From Osler, Sir W.: Aequanimitas with other addresses, 2, Philadelphia, 1930, Blakiston, p. 38.

sible for a decision maker faced with a choice. In these cases application of a decision rule may be what saves the day. If so, the decision maker must be careful to clearly state the grounds for making a decision which may not exactly square with the analysis of alternatives which has taken considerable time and energy. If the decision maker has carefully thought through all stages of the problem, there should be no major discrepancy between intuitive feelings and the results of systematic decision analysis.

Sources of decision rules

Decision rules can be derived from many sources. Normative behavior may be one source for decision rules that can be applied in nursing management.* Hospital administrative policy manuals may be another source for decision rules that will affect the final choice of alternatives. For example, if a hospital policy indicates that employees who violate policies must be reprimanded in writing before punitive action is taken, alternatives that fail to follow this directive should not be selected. Another source of decision rules is a person's own perceptions, personal predilections, and beliefs. What may be a rational decision rule for one person may appear highly irrational to another person whose personal orientation is different.

An organizational hierarchy may be another source for decision rules. Bureaucratic organizations that emphasize tight lines of authority and a rigid charge command tend to preclude certain alternatives fostered by a matrix organization in which persons having special knowledge or skills are assigned to work on specific tasks irrespective of position status within the organization.

FACTORS TO CONSIDER IN APPLYING A DECISION RULE
Two major types of decision rules

As discussed in Chapter 7, there are two basic categories of decision rules: (1) the *satisficing approach,* which attempts to find the first available alternative that will meet the needs or criteria established; and (2) the *optimizing approach,* which intends to find the best alternative among several that have been carefully analyzed.

There are a number of other considerations that must be made when selecting a choice or decision rule. One of these considerations arises from the conditions surrounding the evaluation of the problem itself; others are related to the particular methodology used in analyzing the alternatives.

Accountability

When a decision will affect many contending and vocal interest groups, the choice of an alternative may be subject to attack. Often organizational decision makers get into trouble when they make a decision based upon criteria and goals that may run counter to the goals and intents of the community. For example, if a hospital has chosen to expand its physical facilities rather than move to a new site and if additional property is needed for the expansion, some residents of the neighborhood may object to selling their homes, others may object to the increased traffic, and others may be concerned because they were not involved in the decision making process.

A common pitfall of decision makers is to keep the details of the decision making process secret. The Watergate investigation exemplifies a case in which the stakes of

---

*A norm is a standard of behavior that has been developed over a long period of time or is consistent among a large group of people.

disclosure were high yet secrecy was impossible because it was important to know what decision rules were utilized when a particular operation was authorized. Since decisions often need to be defended, part of the defense is based on the decision rules that were formulated and used in the choice of a certain alternative. This is particularly important in complying with affirmative action programs.

Comprehensibility

When a final choice is made, the choice should be comprehensible to the decision maker's clientele or the people who will be affected by the decision. A decision should be clearly stated and effectively communicated. When there are clear statements of decisions and when decision statements are effectively communicated to everyone concerned, implementation of the decision is less likely to meet with resistance or sabotage.

Urgency

At times decision makers may be pressured to reach early decisions. In such cases it may become necessary to use simpler methods of choosing alternatives even though they are not as comprehensive. Simple procedures (such as the matrix form presented in Chapter 10) that are systematic and logical can provide the decision maker with necessary rationale for a decision action.

Flexibility

Over a long sequence of decision making such as that exemplified during strikes, a decision rule that may be applicable during one time sequence may have to be modified at a later time during negotiations. In such cases it is important that the decision maker be aware that changes will necessitate flexibility in sequential decision making situations.

SELECTING DECISION RULES
Making the best choice

Decision rules do not protect the decision maker against the possibility of making a poor decision. Some decision rules may be so conservative that they rule out effective alternatives in favor of safe alternatives. The decision maker must consider high values as well as risks or safety in formulating decision rules.

Leniency versus severity. Decision rules can be placed on a continuum from leniency to severity. Some rules are punitive and harsh. Such rules place low worth on quantities until very high scores are obtained. On the other end of the continuum are decision rules that are tolerant of low scores and tend to give high worth to quantities that are low or moderate. Decision makers who have plotted a utility curve (see Chapter 10) for each decision criterion can obtain an idea as to whether or not their decision rule is severe or lenient. Curves that bend away with respect to the origin of the graph, that is, the 0 point, tend toward the severity end of the continuum. The degree of severity is roughly proportional to the amount of curvature. Decision rules which are concave, that is, which bend toward the origin, tend toward the leniency pole of the continuum. Again, the degree of leniency is roughly proportional to the amount of curvature. This is illustrated in Fig. 11-1.

In grading student papers or examinations, the effect of two types of utility curves presented in Fig. 11-1, A, can be examined. On the lenient curve, a score of 50 would give the student an A. On the severe curve, a score of 50 would be a failure. In severity curves, low scores of low quantities are penalized and high worth (or utility) scores are

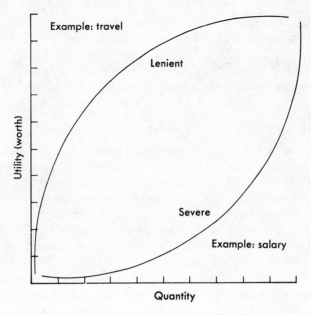

Fig. 11-1. Examples of lenient and severe utility functions (curves).

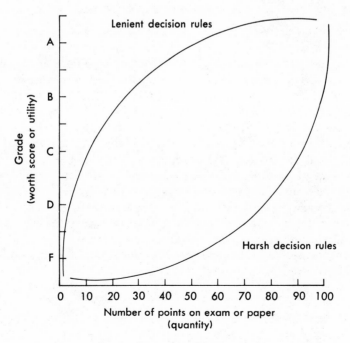

Fig. 11-2. The effects of lenient and severe decision rules on student examination grades.

very difficult to obtain. Fig. 11-2 illustrates the effects of lenient or severe decision rules on student grades.

COMMONLY USED DECISION RULES

There are a number of decision rules that can be utilized. We will not go into many here. The reader is referred to other sources that describe decision rules in more detail.[1,2]

Accept if standards are met

A common satisficing type of decision is to establish a standard of acceptability for each decision criterion and to reject alternatives with scores that fail to meet or exceed those standards. A decision rule of this type is known as a "go/no-go" rule. The standards can be maximum or minimum limits or a combination of the two.

When using a go/no-go type of rule, the criteria must have identical standards. Possible outcomes when using this decision rule are: (1) one alternative will survive the test; (2) no alternatives will survive the test; (3) two or more alternatives will survive the test. If only one alternative survives the test, the problem has been solved. If no alternatives survives, then the decision maker must continue to search for alternatives until one that passes the test is found. An alternative approach is to progressively lower the standards by small increments until one alternative falls into the modified standards. In the latter procedure, standards for less important criteria should be relaxed more rapidly that those having greater weight. The reverse procedure can be used if two or more alternative survive the test, that is, standards can be raised progressively until only one alternative survives. The standards for the more important criteria should be raised more rapidly.

Accept the highest scoring alternative on the criteria which are most important

Decision makers sometimes establish standards of acceptability for every criterion measure except the one that is judged the most important. On this criterion, which is considered a major attribute or major variable, the decision maker makes no decision until all the alternatives have been rejected or accepted by the other criteria. Alternatives that have not been rejected on other criteria are then compared to this criterion measure, and the one with the highest score is judged to be the best alternative to choose.

Accept the alternative with the highest weighted sum score

A procedure used in the grading of certain types of licensing examinations or in computing cumulative grade point averages is a rule that says to select the alternative with the highest weighted-sum score. To obtain this score, the worth scores earned by an alternative on each criterion are multiplied by the corresponding criterion weight.* The resulting products are summed for each alternative. The alternative with the highest weighted sum score is judged to be the best, and the next largest the next best, and so forth. The weighted sum score rule utilizes a combination of both ranking and weighting procedures.

Choose the alternative which is closest to the ideal

Another choice rule is to choose the alternative which is closest to the ideal, that is, the one that has the smallest deviation from the best possible consequences. For example,

---

*Chapter 10 discusses the procedure for obtaining criterion weights.

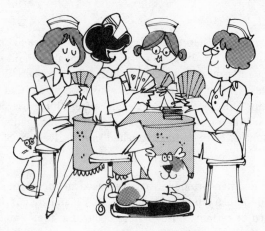

Fig. 11-3. In nursing there are situations which require that decisions be made under conditions of risk or uncertainty.

when a company is looking for a given type of person to take charge of a division or step into a particular type of management job, personality tests may be administered to the candidates and the applicant whose profile is closest to the standard may be chosen, other things being equal.

DECISION RULES OR PRINCIPLES THAT ARE USED WHEN THERE IS RISK OR UNCERTAINTY

In the previous section decision rules were discussed which could be used in planning decisions or in selecting alternatives that meet certain standards. In nursing, there are situations which require that decisions be made under conditions of risk or uncertainty.

The expected value principle is used when risk is involved.* Estimating the expected utility or worth of various consequences of a selected alternative characterizes this principle. The expected value (EV) decision principle tells the decision maker to select the alternative that has the maximum expected value. Since this principle is applied only in situations of risk, it is commonly utilized in health care delivery situations, especially in emergency situations. In these cases, the health professional wants to minimize risk and legal action by selecting an alternative that is expected to have the highest payoff both for the patient and for the health professional.

Two types of value

The expected value (EV) principle is commonly used in decision theory and involves two types of value: (1) *objective value,* which is usually money or some variable of measurable quantity; and (2) *subjective value,* which is called utility. We consider utility to refer to subjective as well as objective quantities since psychologically there are subjective values placed on varying amounts of a commodity. That is, more money is not always "better." For further discussion of utility functions, refer to Chapter 10.

---

*This principle is often called Bayes' theorem after an English mathematician. Presently there is no textbook on Bayesian statistics, and most of the discussions rely heavily on mathematics. Bayes' theorem has been used extensively in computer aided medical diagnosis.[3]

Maximin principle

The maximin decision rule tells the decision maker to choose the alternative having the maximum gain for the smallest risk. In probability and statistics, the maximin principle is frequently used as a decision principle. For each alternative there is a range of consequences. One of the consequences will be worst, that is, it will have the smallest payoff or gain. This becomes the basis for determining the highest gain.

Minimax. When losses are considered rather than gains, the strategy is to minimize the maximum losses that are anticipated from a given set of alternative actions.

Laplace principle

Another decision principle that was used in the early days of probability theory is known as the Laplace principle, named after a statistician. If there is uncertainty about the likelihood of certain consequences occurring, then equal probabilities are assumed. The rule is to choose the option or alternative having the highest mean gain or payoff, given equal likelihoods of occurrence.

Minimax regret

The Minimax regret principle is another decision rule utilized by decision makers. This decision rule tends to minimize the "second thoughts" or regrets that a decision maker would have if an option is chosen which is not the best. Nurses frequently choose the safest option but one that may not be the highest value for the patient, as illustrated in a study of decision making patterns of undergraduate nurses enrolled in a baccalaureate program in a large university.[4] In this study, student nurses were given a simulated problem solving test which required them to make decisions about the care of a patient with a spinal cord injury. Decisions were rated on their general patient care value (high, medium, or low), on the level of the decision (complexity concerning professional nursing actions), and on the amount of risk (high, medium, or low) that was involved. The majority of students tended to select alternatives that had low risk, moderate value, and were in the lower to moderate levels of the decision making process.

REFERENCES

1. Easton, A.: Complex managerial decisions involving multiple objectives, New York, 1973, John Wiley & Sons, Inc.
2. Lee, W.: Decision theory and human behavior, New York, 1971, John Wiley & Sons, Inc.
3. Lusted, L. B.: Introduction to medical decision making, Springfield, Ill., 1968, Charles C Thomas, Publisher.
4. McIntyre, H. M., McDonald, F. J., Bailey, J. T., and Claus, K. E.: The development of a simulated clinical nursing test to assess problem solving behavior of baccalaureate students, Nurs. Res. **21:**429-435, 1972.
5. Osler, Sir W.: Aequanimitas with other addresses, ed. 2, Philadelphia, 1930, Blakiston.

SUGGESTED READING

Brubaker, D. L., and Nelson, R. H., Jr.: Creative survival in educational bureaucracies, Berkeley, Calif., 1974, McCutchan Publishing Corp.

*The effects of the final decision are controlled by taking
other actions to prevent possible adverse consequences from
becoming problems and by making sure the actions decided
on are carried out.*

C. H. KEPNER AND B. B. TREGOE*

> Control
> and
> implement
> decisions

12 IMPLEMENTING THE DECISION

"Making sure the actions are carried out" is the responsibility of a manager. The assumption of this book has been that all nurses are managers to some extent, whether or not their formal title designates this responsibility. Implementing a decision requires the full range of management skills. In nursing, implementing a decision usually requires the blending of activities of many levels of health care services and personnel.

THE PROCESS OF IMPLEMENTING A DECISION

The process of implementing a decision can be compared to a wheel having five major spokes (Fig. 12-1). Implementation involves the following major management functions: (1) planning; (2) organizing; (3) staffing; (4) leading or directing; and (5) controlling. These functions, like the spokes of a wheel, are interrelated, continuous, and interdependent. When carrying out the actions to implement a decision, if one spoke is broken or missing, the wheel is weakened and its purpose thwarted. During the *planning* phase of implementing a decision, realistic objectives, policies, procedures, and strategies need to be carefully considered and selected. *Organizing* involves helping personnel to understand the decision and the procedures for implementing the decision. *Staffing* involves deciding who should assist in carrying out the tasks and when they should be done, that is, selecting the right people for the right job. Once the people are selected for the task, *leadership* and *direction* need to be provided to activate the decision. The *controlling* function is central to implementation. It involves manipulating the environment in such a way that groups within the total system can accomplish the task of activating the decision. The element of control gives the decision a fair chance of being effectively implemented by ensuring that there is sufficient manpower, time, money, supplies, and equipment to accomplish the tasks.

PLANNING

After a decision is made, action must be preceded by thorough and imaginative planning. Carefully developed plans will assist nurses to design action strategies which

---

*From Kepner, C. H., and Tregoe, B. B.: The rational manager, New York, 1965, McGraw-Hill Book Co., p. 50.

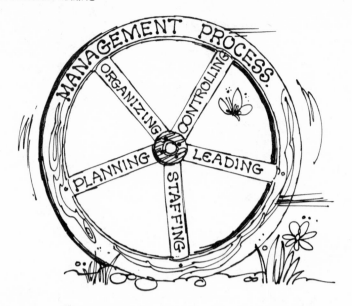

Fig. 12-1. The wheel of implementation.

will support a decision. Strategic planning involves establishing policies and procedures that are needed to implement a decision. Since a managerial decision has impact on a number of claimant groups, implementation plans must be practical and flexible. Implementation planning involves five major areas: policies, procedures, budgeting, scheduling, and promoting ideas.

Policies

Policies are types of plans designed to reinforce goals and objectives. In essence, they guide thinking by providing directions for those who are responsible for implementing a decision. Policies provide common premises for action to assist in the coordination of effort.

In implementing a decision, nurses are responsible for making policies clear to all groups within the total system. Shared understanding fosters effective interpersonal relationships and teamwork.

Policies provide common grounds for action, and assist nurses to delegate authority and to involve others at various management levels. Without the involvement of the various management levels of nursing, there is no assurance that there will be consistent handling of problems that could arise in the implementation process.

Principles of use. Five principles that are helpful in the development of implementation policies are: (1) the policy should be consistent with higher level policy; (2) policies should help clarify decision objectives; (3) statement of policies should be broad enough to permit discretionary action by responsible personnel; (4) subordinate personnel involved in implementing the decision should understand, support, and apply new policies; and, (5) policies should form an adequate basis for delegating authority and for decentralizing the organizational structure.

Procedures

Procedures are types of plans which specify how a task should be performed. In essence, procedures are guides for action. Procedures save time by making it unnecessary for personnel to try to devise ways to do a task well; thus procedures can be used to prevent costly errors in implementation.

Workers who are engaged in repetitive tasks do not have to decide how a job will be done if procedures are developed which allow them to concentrate on accuracy and speed of performance. Procedures also foster consistency and uniformity in the quality of work and utilize the specialized talents or expertise of each member of the health care team. Experts can determine the best way to perform particular tasks and teach the procedure to others.

When to have standard procedures. Standard operating procedures are helpful when the following conditions exist: (1) the given tasks are repetitive and must be done frequently by several people; (2) there are potential hazards to personnel or equipment if proper procedures are not observed; and (3) unacceptable levels of nursing care would yield significant losses or risks.

Budgeting

A budget is a plan for the allocation of resources to achieve a decision objective. A budget simply states expected results expressed in numbers. The statement can be financial (expenses, revenues, capital budgets), or nonfinancial (materials, equipment or output per person). For a manager, a budget can aid control by ensuring that results conform to plans. The purpose of a budget is to help the manager determine what resources should be expended by whom, where, and for what.

Types of budgets. Nurses in a management position will generally deal with three or four categories of budgets. *Operating expense budgets* deal primarily with salaries of personnel, supplies, and contractual services. *Time, material, product,* or *space budgets* are nonfinancial in nature but can usually be translated into dollar values. Such budgets may be comprised of instructor hours, nurse-patient interaction hours, equipment hours, units of material, square feet of floor space, man hours or man days of work.

Equipment and *facilities expense budgets,* often called *capital expense budgets,* concern requests for new equipment facilities or replacements. Capital expenditures have dollar values that have been fixed and that have a relatively long life expectancy. Physical plant improvements, furniture, and major medical equipment fall into this category. Long-term planning and commitment for extended use over a period of time are necessary when capital expense budgets are being considered.

Cash budgets forecast cash receipts and disbursements. This type of budget is devised to ensure that cash is available to meet financial obligations when they come due. Budgeting of this type is important for nurses engaged in private practice who often rent office space in carrying out their practice.

In summary, the budget is a means of expressing the philosophy, goals, and objectives of the decision maker. The budget is influenced by the orientation of the organization as well as of the decision maker. Public and private institutions such as hospitals are usually input-oriented because their income is derived from admission fees and other initial income. Charges for rooms and other fees are frequently increased to keep pace with inflation, salary increases of personel, and costs of living in general.

Scheduling

A practical part of implementation consists of scheduling. Realistic and workable schedules are paramount in implementing decisions. Scheduling ensures smooth implementation of a decision.

Types of schedules. Three basic types of schedules can be utilized: (1) simple projects require a straightforward listing of critical steps and target completion dates; (2) complex projects may require block diagrams and possible a flow chart; and (3) highly complex projects involving many different agencies and levels of personnel may necessitate network schedules such as those used by government agencies.* The type of schedule selected will depend upon time resources and the number of personnel available.

"Selling" ideas within the organization

Nursing need to identify people within the organization who have an interest in implementing a decision once it has been made. They need to sell their ideas. To be saleable, decisions should accomplish results as a reasonable cost. Results usually refer to desired behavioral changes that are measurable in terms of job or task performance. Methods for measuring results and treatment of data must be reliable and reproduceable. Presentations of data indicating results need to be clear, concise, and appealing. The format of an idea, that is, how it appears at its presentation, has a direct bearing on its saleability.

The selling process incorporates such techniques as underscoring the results achieved by the new decision; presenting data on improvements in patient care, improvements in personnel policies, or cost reduction; and other objective evidence relative to effectively presenting the results.

ORGANIZING

The process of implementing a decision involves elements of organizing for efficiency and effectiveness. For example, a decision cannot be properly implemented if information is given to one group of employees and not to others. Organizing implies that plans have been carefully made and carried out so that all groups within a system understand the decision and how it will affect them. Since nursing managers cannot personally perform all the duties and tasks required to implement a managerial decision, some tasks must be assigned to subordinates together with the authority needed to carry out the tasks.

The elements of an organization plan provide a framework within which a group can work together to attain the goals and objectives of the decision. It is a means of ensuring opportunities for coordination of the activities of the personnel who will be involved in implementation. By identifying functions and activities, by grouping and assigning capable persons to given tasks, the nurse manager can better ensure that implementation procedures will be effective.

There are certain organizational dysfunctions that nurse mangers should recognize: inadequate job descriptions that fail to define duties clearly; unclear lines of authority, which require a person to report to more than one supervisor; illogical work assignments, which fail to use the competencies and skills of the individual; and dead-end jobs, which do not provide opportunity for personal growth and development. Each one of these problems may be faced by nurse managers as they deal with organizing and implementing decisions.

The nurse manager who is interested in implementing a managerial decision needs to consider five major aspects of organizing the effort: (1) grouping, (2) assigning duties and delegating authority; (3) charting and graphing; (4) job descriptions; and (5) data collection.

---

*Program Evaluation and Review Techniques, called PERT for short, are common in the military and it is not unusual for armed service nurses to be responsible for meeting PERT schedules.

Grouping

The nurse manager must be able to group needed implementation functions and activities into logical subdivisions. Several bases are appropriate for grouping activities: number, function, process, product, location, time, and patient.

The nurse manager should give special attention to two factors as grouping assignments are made: *specialization* and *span of management*. Specialization refers to groupings of individuals with highly specialized skills. No one individual, regardless of experience and education, will be able to possess all the skills required in the delivery of health care. Clinical nurse specialists exemplify one type of grouping assignment. Span of management refers to how many subordinates a manager can supervise. The number of persons supervised should be kept to a minimum.

Assigning duties and delegating authority

Nurses assign duties and delegate authority to persons subordinate to them in the organizational structure. As a rule, authority should be delegated as far down the organization as is possible.[7]

Certain guidelines are useful for the proper delegation of authority:

1. If a person is to be held accountable for performance, enough authority must also be delegated to do the job.
2. Routine and recurring jobs and tasks should be delegated.
3. Jobs that are the concern of only one subordinate should be delegated to that subordinate.
4. Nurse managers should retain authority to take actions that involve two or more subordinates or involve persons outside their particular department or unit.

Organizational charts and graphs

An organizational chart depicts the formal relationships within an organization by graphically portraying the component parts in those relationships. Major considerations in chart arrangement are its completeness, simplicity, clarity, symmetry, and unity. The name of the organization or group should appear at the bottom of the chart, with the date when the chart was devised. Too much information on one chart should be avoided. Fig. 12-2 illustrates the right and wrong ways to construct a simple ward unit chart.

Clarity and simplicity are not synonymous. Simplicity implies a small number of organizational components or blocks and a small number of lines joining the blocks. But if lines are confused or blocks are not labeled, the chart lacks clarity.

Developing job descriptions

The nurse manager is responsible for formulating written job descriptions for each position in the structure as a means of defining the duties, functions, and authorities assigned to a given position. A job description should specify the functions and major duties of a job, the scope of authority, and the relationships between the position and other positions in the department and the organization. Job descriptions inform people of what they are expected to do and what they will be held accountable for doing.

Collecting relevant data

Nurse managers should be responsible for collecting adequate data that will enable them to implement decisions.[1, 8] Several methodologies of data collection can be utilized: records, questionnaires, interviews, observation, and measurement.

A CONFUSED WARD CHART

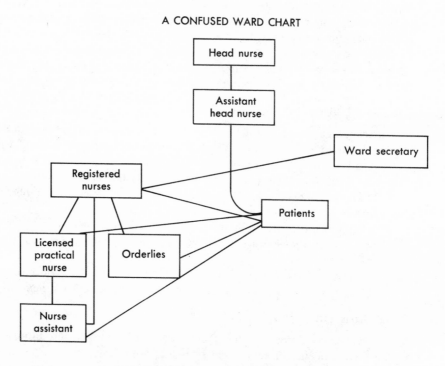

A MORE CONCISE WAY TO DIAGRAM A WARD

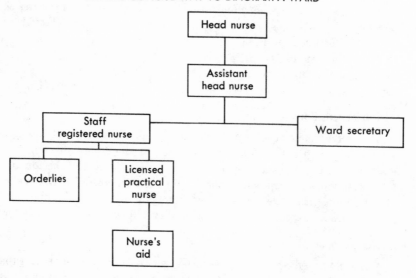

Fig. 12-2. An example of an organizational chart which has been simplified for clarity.

Records. Existing records provide background information that is useful in evaluating the effectiveness of the problem solving decision action. Records such as policies, instructions, procedure manuals, statistical reports, and correspondence can be studied by using documentary analysis techniques.[4] The nurse manager is cautioned, however, never to draw conclusions from records alone.

Questionnaires. Use of a questionnaire is a basic data-collection technique designed to solicit information from personnel and consumers. If questionnaires are properly designed and administered, they can yield valuable information for use in evaluating the effectiveness of a decision action.

Interviews. Interviews are not a substitute for other data-gathering techniques, but should be used as a supplemental procedure. They are an effective method for gathering information to clarify responses to questionnaires. Both interviewer and interviewee tend to be motivated by the process. Face-to-face contact often assists people to recall facts that would otherwise not have occurred to them, or which they may be reticent to divulge in writing. The interviewer should know in advance what information is wanted and how to go about getting it. Interview sessions should be kept informal and limited to information gathering. The tape recorder can be used to record the interviewing sessions although the procedure is costly and time-consuming and may cause the interviewee to become uneasy. The interviewer may prefer to take notes. Whatever procedure is used, a written record should be made of the information given.

Observation. Another method of gathering facts is direct observation. Nurses are effective observers of patients and observation is used extensively in direct patient care activities. Observation has limitations in fact finding because it is costly and time consuming.

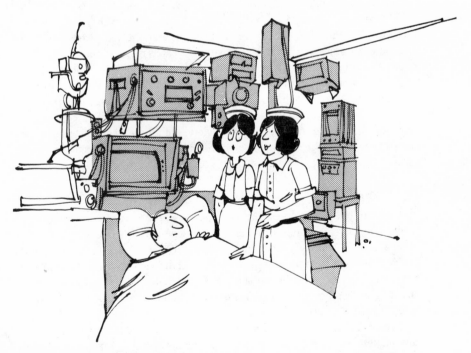

Fig. 12-3. There's really nothing to C.C.U., Miss Jones.

Measurement. In health care delivery settings, numerous machines and monitors are used to obtain specific measurements of patients' conditions. Other measurement devices used by management personnel include personality tests, attitude inventories, job orientation or preference indices, and other standardized tests.

The necessity for nurse input

It is important to have nursing input in making staffing decisions. Nurse managers are responsible for implementing staffing decisions and for ensuring that high-quality patient care is maintained. Sometimes staffing decisions and goals of quality patient care run at cross purposes. For example, staffing intensive care units or coronary care units with staff nurses who have no specialized training may be expedient but may place considerable added responsibility on experienced clinical nurse specialists on the same units. The combination of inexperience and lack of specialized training on one side and overwork on the other may seriously threaten the quality of patient care.

The very situation described above was the basis for a professional nurses strike in June, 1974 in forty-three hospitals in northern California. Four thousand nurses made sacrifices during 3 weeks of bargaining and mediation to achieve the right to have a significant voice in hospital staffing. The element of staffing is an important dimension of management and a critical factor in the implementation of a decision. The nurse manager must give careful attention to staffing when changes are made in the work environment (such as the 4-day–40-hour week); adjustments will be required in staffing patterns and providing nursing services.

Job turnover

A perennial problem in maintaining a competent staff is the rate of job turnover. Generally, there are two opposing trends in the nurse work force. First, there is an increase in the level of education for one group of nurses with a high level of training and expert skill. These nurses are willing to assume greater responsibility, and accordingly they demand more opportunities for self-direction and self-determination. On the other hand, there is an increase in the number of nurses who have aspirations for better jobs and opportunities to achieve their dreams but who characteristically have lower levels of education and who may lack knowledge of certain skills. The challenge of the nurse manager is to utilize the skills and knowledge of all members of the staff in meeting the goals and needs of the organization as well as meeting the needs and goals of the nursing staff.

DIRECTING AND LEADING

Probably one of the most critical functions of management is leading and directing others. Effective leadership and direction depends on effective personal relationships between nurse manager and subordinates. The key to effective leadership is to get people to perform well their required tasks and duties, not to avoid reprimand and punishment, but because they get satisfaction from a job well done. In other words, the art of directing or leading is the art of influencing others in such a way that they will work to achieve goals because they *want* to, not because they *have* to.

Effective directing or leadership involves the coordination or integration of several complementary techniques: motivating; communicating; appraising and counseling; building and maintaining morale.

Motivating others

Motivation comes from experiences such as being assigned to stimulating work, having considerable responsibility, and being given assignments of some importance. A key to sustaining motivation seems to lie in assignments that push individuals to the limits of their abilities, but not beyond—assignments that match gross abilities and skills with new and bigger challenges.[5]

Motivation of nurse professionals is not determined exclusively by deeply ingrained personal needs. Ideas and values shared with other professionals also serve as motivators. Values result from educational and cultural experiences to which professional nurses have been exposed throughout their careers. Professional norms and standards determine to a large extent what professional nurses do, say, and think.

A few general guidelines may prove helpful to the manager in building and maintaining motivation:

1. Develop a supportive organizational environment.
2. Lower the potential for failure.
3. Reduce the physical stress associated with the job.
4. Coordinate personal and organizational needs.
5. Provide opportunities for self-expression.
6. Provide recognition.
7. Provide feedback to help a person evaluate his own performance.
8. Make clear the expectation of the role or job assigned.

Communicating with subordinates

Communication is among the most critical of the implementation processes. Facts, ideas, opinions, beliefs, and feelings are exchanged among human beings in the work environment through communication networks. Nurses need to deal with verbal and nonverbal expression and semantics as well as written communications. They also need to be aware of how people within the organization may facilitate, block, or distort communication.

Purposes of communication. The purposes of communication for the nurse manager are threefold: (1) to provide staff members with the information and the understanding needed to attain goals and objectives; (2) to assist the nurse manager to use information for building teamwork and for furthering job satisfaction of staff members; and (3) to provide staff members with guidance, assistance, encouragement, and feedback on performance.

A leader must not assume that communication essentially means telling or giving information. *Telling* a person to do something will rarely produce the results expected—telling is only a part of effective communication. Other processes of equal importance are: *questioning* to obtain additional information; *listening* in an interested, careful way; and *understanding* the communication, the most important process of all.

The communication process. Fig. 12-4 uses a systems framework to illustrate the sequence of events in the communication process. Basically, communication is interaction between a communicator and a receiver. Nurse managers can develop more effective communication if they think in terms of three basic elements in both communicator and receiver systems: input, throughput, and output. The communicator starts with an idea, puts it into words (or other symbols), and sends it to the intended receiver. The receiver perceives what he thinks the message said, interprets it, and acts on his interpretation. When writing reports, speaking to superiors or subordinates, or giving a

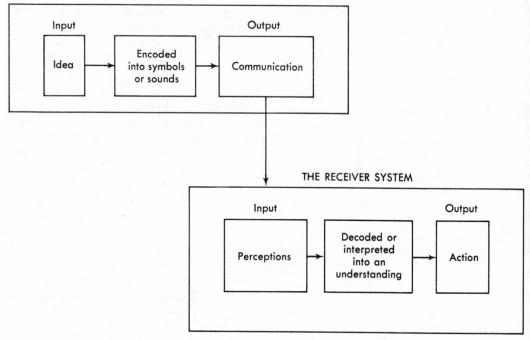

Fig. 12-4. The process of communication seen as the interaction between communicator and receiver systems.

lecture (or any other type of communication), it is helpful in planning the presentation to think in terms of the six elements shown in Fig. 12-4.

1. What is the idea you wish to express?
2. In what form do you wish to express it?
3. How can you ensure that the intended receiver will hear or see it?
4. How do you think the receiver will perceive the message?
5. Will the receiver understand what you mean?
6. Will the receiver act upon your communication? (And does the action indicate that the message was understood?)

Barriers to communication. The nurse manager should be wary of certain recurring problems or barriers to communication. If objectives are inappropriate or unrealistic, they may not be accepted by staff members. There may be a credibility gap, that is, the communicators may not be trusted. The nurse manager must guard against an organizational climate of distrust, conflict, animosity, or anxiety. A work environment characterized by distrust and anxiety will reduce the amount of information flow and cause people to block, screen, or distort communication. Communication practices are strongly influenced by the rewards and penalties that subordinates experience. When penalities are imposed, communication channels tend to dry up. Only information that is safe is passed on.

Another barrier to communication is organizational distance; that is, when organizational levels are widely different and people at different levels have different perspectives or ways of thinking, communication may be ineffective. Barriers of social distance can be surmounted if communicators are able to put themselves in the position of receivers when they are framing or sending messages (see Fig. 12-4).

Rules for effective communication. Rules for effective communication, regardless of format are the following.

1. Clarity: avoid unfamiliar words or jargon, which might confuse the receiver.
2. Brevity: use only one idea in a sentence; short communications are easier to understand.
3. Simplicity: every word should count; avoid extra words.
4. Precision: words that have a standard or universal meaning should be used.
5. Integrity: communication is a *means,* not an end; its purpose is to pass on information and enhance understanding; avoid forcing receiver to "read between the lines."
6. Specificity: channels of communication between positions (not persons) should be clear.
7. Continuity: the complete chain of command should usually be used.
8. Directness: the shorter, more direct the line of communication, the greater the speed and the smaller the probability of error.
9. Completeness: everyone should have a definite line of communication within the organization.
10. Openness: lines of communication should remain open, that is, someone should occupy each critical point at all times so that information can reach those who need it.

Appraising and counselling

In implementing a decision, the nurse manager is often called upon to appraise the performance and potential of subordinate workers in terms of overall effectiveness, strengths and weakness in knowledge and skills, and whether or not responsibilities can be expanded. Hand in hand with appraisal goes the task of counselling subordinates in the areas of future training and development needs, progress toward personal goals and objectives, readiness for new jobs or for promotion, and motivation and growth. Both appraisal and counselling utilize decision making skills. Appraisal depends upon systematic comparison of performance with goals or standards. Counselling is a one-to-one problem solving process in which feedback on performance appraisal is often the starting point for action. Both processes require objectivity, a direct approach (no beating about the bush), patience and tact, continuous effort, and a helping, cooperative attitude.

A few pointers to aid the nurse manager in effective appraisal are: (1) schedule periodic appraisal; (2) establish performance standards cooperatively with employee; and (3) be fair, objective, and systematic.

Counselling is often considered an art because it concerns large areas which are emotionally charged, especially when personal problems are involved. The nurse manager should not attempt to deal with sensitive issues unless specially trained to do so. There are some ground rules, however, for effective counseling sessions: (1) arrange the environment so that it is private, orderly, free of distractions, and comfortable; (2) avoid a sense of haste; allow enough time; (3) prepare—examine records and other information prior to the session.

Building and maintaining morale

Implementing a decision may require high levels of performance. Such performance occurs when people are motivated to do their best. Positively motivated people usually have high morale. Morale refers to attitude—how a person or a group feels about the things that affect and are important to them.

Since morale is a variable that affects performance, it is helpful for the nurse charged with implementing a decision to consider how morale can be built and maintained. Most people react to other people, things, ideas, and situations in characteristic, predictable ways. This consistency of action and attitude gives a person his particular "character" and colors how that person perceives the world. A person's experiences encourage certain expectations about what will happen. Many times employees feel mistreated or discouraged because they have developed expectations about their job that cannot be fulfilled.

Factors affecting morale. The nurse manager can examine two major categories of sources of satisfaction or dissatisfaction in evaluating morale: job environment factors and motivational factors.[2,6] Job factors include physical, social, and security factors. Motivational factors include attitudes that correspond to an individual's need hierarchy; achievement, acceptance, responsibility, recognition, growth.

Some pointers. The nurse manager can take the following steps to build and maintain morale:

1. Develop a system to keep informed about new knowledge and pass new findings on to staff.
2. Determine the level of morale and pinpoint areas of dissatisfaction.
3. Develop and make public policies that use human resources.
4. Develop ways to measure the motivating effects of policies and procedures.
5. Reward successful performance.

CONTROLLING

"The best laid plans of mice and men . . ." Plans can indeed be sabotaged without the effective control of human and material resources within the total health care system. Control should be designed to reflect the structure and character of the decision action through the use of realistic and measurable standards. Subjective standards are preferable to no standards at all; however, some quantitative description should be applied.

The controlling procedure should detect potential deviations from the plan and should allow a minimum of unanticipated results. Effective control does not leave room for major surprises. Prompt feedback should be a product of control.

Although control goes hand in hand with effective planning, ineffective control can lead personnel away from plans. There may be a gradual lowering of standards or a gradual changing of conditions which may not be perceived until management recognizes that the desired performance level is not being achieved. Nurse managers who recognize the importance of control will not delegate the authority to others for controlling the environment.

Approaches to control

Nurse managers can employ two general approaches to control in the implementation stage. They can directly and *personally execute control* based on personal observation, or they can *develop guidelines and procedures* to identify variances in performance or failure of results. For example, establishing too many controls should be avoided, as an inordinate number of controls stifle creativity and work satisfaction; controls that are excessively detailed are confusing and frustrating; and controls that are used as a means of enforcing rules and procedures detract from the primary function of control, which is to attain objectives and produce results.

Types of control measures

Four types of effective control measures that the nurse manager can utilize are discussed in the following paragraphs.

Quality control. Quality control is the systematic control of variables that affect an end product. Quality control measures follow established standards.*

Manpower control. One of the most effective ways to control human resources is through the establishment of proper and realistic performance standards. Identification of deviations from those standards and correction of the deviations are controlling methods. Guidelines that promote effective control procedures include: carefully defining the objectives; clearly delineating the area to be controlled; precisely defining performance, such as the desired nurse-patient ratios for particular units or areas; determining deviations from standards; and reviewing and auditing the control system periodically to ensure that needed changes are made.

Cost control. Although nurse managers may not be directly responsible for cost control, they should aim to optimize the operation of the nursing service, unit, or department through the identification, analysis, and control of major cost components. Such cost components include manpower, materials, supplies, utilities, equipment, maintenance, travel, consultants, and other components for meeting patient care and employee needs.

Budget control. Nurse managers will probably be accountable for a balanced budget, although they may delegate the details of the task of monitoring and regulating the budget to an administrative assistant. Budget controls and adequate knowledge of budgetary matters reassure both superiors and subordinates that the nurse manager is concerned with this important area of resource allocation.

In summary, effective controls must be understandable, timely, appropriate, adequate, flexible, diagnostic, objective, and economical. To assist the nurse manager to develop an effective control system, the following guidelines are presented:

1. Identify key or critical functions and activities—those activities that make the difference between success and failure.
2. Collect and assemble all available data on the activity.
3. Analyze the data and find out at which point important actions take place.
4. Identify or consider alternative means of control, such as procedures and regulatory measures, organizational changes, revision or establishment of records and reports.
5. Install new control systems incrementally and on a trial basis if possible.
6. Analyze the results achieved by a new system.
7. Modify the system as required and install changes.

Effective control measures establish reasonable and objectively measurable standards, using these standards to measure progress and performance, evaluating progress and performance, and finally, correcting deviations from performance standards.

---

*See Chapter 15.

REFERENCES

1. Abdellah, F. G., and Levine, E.: Better patient care through nursing research, New York, 1965, The Macmillan Co.
2. Hughes, C. L.: Goal setting: key to individual and organizational effectiveness, New York, 1965, American Management Association.
3. Kepner, C. H., and Tregoe, B. B.: The rational manager, New York, 1965, McGraw-Hill Book Co.
4. Kerlinger, F. N.: Foundations of behavioral research; educational and psychological inquiry, New York, 1964, Holt, Rinehart & Winston.
5. Maslow, A.: Motivation and personality, New York, 1954, Harper & Row, Publishers.
6. Myers, M. A.: Every employee a manager: more meaningful work through job enrichment, New York, 1970, McGraw-Hill Book Co.
7. Parkinson, C. N.: Parkinson's law, Boston, 1957, Houghton-Mifflin.
8. Treece, E. W., and Treece, J. W., Jr.: Elements of research in nursing, St. Louis, 1973, The C. V. Mosby Co.

SUGGESTED READING

Zimbardo, P., and Ebbesen, E. B.: Influencing attitudes and changing behavior, (revised printing), Reading, Mass., 1970, Addison-Wesley Publishing Co.

Evaluate
effectiveness
of
action

13 EVALUATING THE EFFECTIVENESS OF A DECISION

The use of criteria and standards to evaluate the effectiveness of an action decision is basically a two-step process. First, criteria and standards must be established (see Chapter 8). Second, a measurement procedure must be developed to sample the results of the decision.

Evaluation serves as a link between the steps in the problem solving process by being the source of feedback data. In a cybernetic system, evaluation is a critical element.

THE IMPORTANCE OF EVALUATION

Evaluation is one of the most important elements of management and implementation (see discussion of control in Chapter 11). Effective evaluation procedures will provide a decision maker with a method to assess the effects of a decision after it has been implemented. Evaluation can also point to areas where it may be necessary to take corrective action. A significant difference between expected standards and the results of a decision after it has been implemented tells the decision maker that there is still a problem. Corrective action can then be taken. This action may involve working through the problem, solving steps again until the discrepancy falls within tolerable limits.

ESTABLISHING STANDARDS

Standards are the criteria against which methods, performance, and results can be measured. They describe the ideal conditions that exist when a job or function is being done effectively, how it must be done, and how well it must be performed. Standards are an objective basis against which to test performance in terms of quality, quantity, timeliness, or cost. Standards are generally broader than decision criteria and serve as a yardstick against which nurse managers and subordinates can evaluate their own performance.

_____
*From Bloom, B.: Taxonomy of educational objectives: the classification of educational goals: Handbook I: cognitive domain, New York, 1965, David McKay Co., p. 185.

Characteristics of good standards

One of the most critical dimensions of a standard is that it should be attainable. Standards should also be objective, reasonable, comprehensible, and acceptable to those who use them. A performance standard should accomplish the following things: (1) identify discrepancies; (2) indicate the need for corrective action; (3) provide a basis for developing meaningful reports of progress.

Types of standards

There are numerous types of standards that can be used to assess the effects of a decision action. General types of standards with which nurses frequently come into contact include: personnel standards; space and facilities standards; equipment standards; material standards; time standards; service standards; patient care or client standards; monetary standards; and cost standards.

Procedures for developing standards

In developing standards, the following steps are helpful:
1. Identify key points in a department or unit where control can be expected.
2. Look for existing standards used in similar situations or institutions.
3. If existing standards cannot be found, seek input from personnel who will be directly involved in the activity or seek the advice of experts.
4. Develop a trial set of standards for each key control point and revise the standards according to input received from reviewers.
5. Try out the standards on a pilot basis and collect and analyze appropriate data.
6. Modify and implement the standards in accordance with the findings.
7. Periodically review and revise the standards.

MEASURING PERFORMANCE BY MEANS OF STANDARDS

Decision makers must be able to measure performance by comparing observed behavior with the standards that have been formulated. Measuring involves the use of personal observation, audits, ratings, tests, surveys, reports, and records.

Personal observation

Personal observation of on-the-job activities is an important means of measuring performance and determining the progress of employees. Observations should be planned and systematic. Nurses need to consider the following in planning observations: (1) who should be observed; (2) what behaviors should be observed; (3) where observations should be made (what units); (4) when the observations should be made (time); (5) how frequently the observations should be made; and (6) how the findings should be used and reported.

Personal or direct observation has three major limitations: subjectivity, the presence of the observer (a variable which may alter the situation), and fragmentary reporting resulting from the problem of observing and recording information at the same time. To avoid this latter difficulty, a sampling technique that involves brief observation at critical points can be used. For example, rapport between nurses and patients or between instructors and students can be observed at critical points in a relatively short period of time.

The audit

Audits are used to assess the adequacy of a procedure when compared against practices and established criteria. There are basically two types of audits used by nurses in

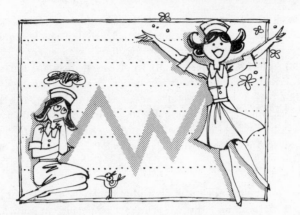

Fig. 13-1. Decision makers must be able to measure performance by comparing observed behavior with the standards that have been formulated.

health settings: quality audits (problem-oriented medical records) and procedures audits (the nursing audit).*

Quality audits are inspections of quality. They are usually planned and scheduled on a periodic basis so that critical practices or procedures can be assessed within an established time frame. Such audits are used to determine whether procedures or products have deteriorated because of personnel turnover, rearrangements of work loads, or new equipment or facilities. Preplanned checklists make possible periodic audits of selected workers or performance areas.

Procedures audits compare ongoing operations against applicable procedures to determine whether documents such as standing orders are current, complete, understood, and used by the personnel involved.

Ratings

Ratings are an attempt to systematize judgments and to remove subjective bias. Ratings are useful when characteristics cannot be measured by tests. There are two basic types of rating methods: relative and absolute.

Relative ratings are used when several persons, situations, or processes are being compared. Common relative rating scales are: (1) *rank order*—members of a group are arranged from best to worst, highest to lowest; (2) *equal intervals*—the rater places individuals in groups that seem to be equally spaced (average, above average, below average); (3) *paired comparisons*—the rater compares each member of a class or group with every other member to obtain a ranking of the entire group. This technique can be used only with relatively small numbers of people or things because of the number of comparisons that must be made. Only one trait or characteristic should be compared at a time.

Absolute rating methods are used when a rater is required to assign absolute values to a performance being measured without reference to the performance of any other person or thing. The rater places the person on a fixed scale. Examples of this type of method are: (1) *numerical scales*, usually utilizing an odd number of points with the middle number representing the average; (2) *descriptive scales*, which use adjectives

---

*See Chapter 15.

or phrases to rate levels of ability or performance; (3) *graphic scales,* which combine numerical and descriptive scales; (4) *checklists,* which require the rater to check the presence or absence of a condition; (5) *forced-choice scales,* which use two to five favorable and unfavorable descriptions from which the rater must select the statement that best describes the person or performance; (6) *critical incidents,* which require the rater to judge a person or performance against a list of statements that describe incidents that have been judged to be of primary importance in the effective performance of a job or operation; and (7) *performance standards,* which require the rater to pass or fail a person on preestablished performance standards for a particular job or task.

Surveys

Surveys, another means of collecting data, can be used for identifying and diagnosing problems, determining the expectations of people, measuring employee attitudes and morale, and determining the status of specific management areas. They call attention to particular aspects of a situation or problem. Surveys can extend the nurse manager's power of observation by standardizing and objectifying the observations. A well-constructed survey instrument specifies the terminology and the units used in reporting the observations, and ensures that responses to the same item are collected from all respondents.

Diagnostic surveys are designed to analyze specific problems or situations. These surveys are conducted to uncover reasons for a problem, to probe feelings about a situation, to get ideas for a solution.

Intentional surveys are designed to complement other means of forecasting. They may be used to identify significant changes in patient expectations or student expectations.

Attitude and morale surveys are designed to detemine the interests, ideas, opinions, problems, and concerns of employees. They are used to improve upward communication. Their ultimate purpose is to help management better understand how to motivate people to work.

Wage and salary rate surveys are used to assist the manager in dealing with important compensation policy matters. These surveys are usually conducted so that comparisons can be made and salaries adjusted if they are found to be lagging.

Tests

Two major types of tests are used in evaluation. One type is associated with plans, procedures, or equipment and its purpose is to determine adequacy, effectiveness, durability, serviceability, and utility of the items or to measure the knowledge of employees about the above factors. The second type of test, the psychological test, is used to classify and group employees, to determine the effectiveness and quality of instructional systems, to provide a basis for guiding and assisting employees, and to keep management informed about progress and results. The results of psychological tests can be used as a basis for personal development if employees are allowed to use results as feedback. For example, in a leadership training program for graduate nurses, students receive computer printouts of their profiles on a number of psychological tests.* Students use this data to plan their own learning experiences. Students also work with staff members in evaluation of

---

*The Creative Leadership Development Program, School of Nursing, University of California, San Francisco (for masters', postmasters' and doctoral students).

progress toward goals which they set for themselves, using pre- and posttest comparisons of their profiles on the psychological tests.

Reports and records

If reports and records are prepared and stored properly, the task of managing becomes easier. Managers must be able to gather information from reports which describe certain activities in their unit. Reports not only provide a continuous check on results for which the nurse manager is accountable, but they also provide a basis for making future plans. Reports can assist the nurse-manager in evaluating and improving performance, especially if they measure results in terms of quality, quantity, speed, accuracy, and cost.

A good reporting system provides measures that are definite and objective. Reports also eliminate confusion that arises from multiplicity of facts, figures, or ideas with regard to a given situation. Reports can provide the data for review and analysis of operations. They can indicate failures or deficiencies and can serve to point the way to corrective action.

Reports are expensive if they are not used or are used improperly. There is often as much danger in too much information as there is in too little information—the right kind of information must be available in a record. A major problem in using a record system, such as the problem oriented medical record, is to balance information against its value.* It is important that the nurse decide in advance what information will be recorded, how often it should be recorded, and how to summarize the information.

EFFECTIVE EVALUATION

Evaluation involves comparing results to standards, reviewing all deviations including those within the tolerances, and applying judgment with respect to the seriousness of the discrepancies and needs for correction. Although performance will not always measure up to the standards, it should come "reasonably close" to matching expectations. The nurse manager must define what is reasonably close.

Guidelines

The following guidelines may be of some assistance in conducting an effective evaluation:

1. Get all relevant facts.
2. Focus on significant variations between the evaluative standards and observed performance (refer back to procedures used in Chapter 5 for defining a problem).
3. Determine the cause of observed discrepancies.
4. Identify alternative approaches to treatment of the discrepancies. For example, are the standards too high or too low? Is the observed deviation important in terms of the decision goals?
5. Examine each approach for likely consequences. For example, would lowering standards affect quality of care?

Evaluation, in essence, is a matter of comparing results with standards and involves application of the problem solving approach. Nurses need to be able to utilize all the steps described earlier in this book in problem solving activities.

---

*See Chapter 15.

Major considerations

In order to be effective, evaluation should be conducted in accordance with accepted and proven principles and procedures. The following are some major considerations that the nurse manager should weigh in a formal evaluation:

1. Evaluation should be *planned in advance;* it cannot be haphazard.
2. Evaluation should be conducted *in terms of objectives and purposes.*
3. Evaluation should be *objective,* based upon uniform and agreed upon standards and procedures.
4. Evaluation should be *verifiable;* its results must be reliable and therefore subject to replication.
5. Evaluation should be *a cooperative effort.* All those who are involved in the operation of a unit should be involved and those affected by the evaluation should participate in the process.
6. Evaluation should be *specific,* pinpointing strengths and weaknesses, achievements and deficiencies.
7. Evaluation should be *quantitative.* This does not preclude qualitative assessment but it does mean that techniques should be utilized which will enable the nurse manager to place quantitative values on subjective worth. (Refer to Chapter 10 and the discussion of assessed worth and utility.)
8. Evaluation should be *feasible.* The evaluation process should not be unmanageable or too costly.
9. Evaluation should *result in useful information.* Products of the evaluation process can and should be used in control of the operation of a unit. Evaluation must elicit necessary information rather than information that merely satisfies curiosity.

PERSPECTIVES OF EVALUATION

There are three complementary and different approaches to evaluation. *Internal evaluation* focuses on ongoing processes in an ongoing program. The major objective of internal evaluation is to assess the quality of operations. Participant reaction is a common method of evaluation from the internal perspective. Measures of behavioral change during the operation is another way to obtain information for internal evaluation. This is often used in an instructional setting in which the evaluation focuses on the measurement of learning that occurs as a direct result of the experiences provided in a training program. Measurements can involve paper and pencil performance tests, observations, ratings, or questioning. The self audit is another technique used to probe the quality of specific aspects of an operation from the viewpoint of selected groups.

External evaluation is used to evaluate results of new programs and usually takes place when employees are on the job. There are usually two classes of external criteria: those related to changes in on-the-job behavior, and those related to changes within the organization.

Intermediate evaluation is often used at the conclusion of special programs or projects. The objective of this type of evaluation is to elicit reactions to the new situations and experiences.

REVIEW AND ANALYSIS OF PROGRESS AND RESULTS

Periodic review and analysis are used to evaluate the efficiency of departments and units in utilizing resources, especially in those areas requiring decision action by a manager. *Review* usually refers to critical examination of an activity to discover achievements and deficiencies at given points during a specified period of time. The emphasis is on critical examination of factual material. *Analysis* is the process of breaking down the activity into component parts. Each part is then studied in relation to other parts or to the whole. The emphasis here is on clarification of facts. Therefore the review and analysis procedure is a critical examination and clarification of facts pertaining to particular problems that require direct managerial decision making. The process of review and analysis usually involves the assembly and analysis of recorded and reported data.

Types of review and analysis

There are two basic types of review and analysis: activity analysis, often called *vertical analysis,* and department-wide analysis, often called *composite analysis.* Vertical review and analysis is performed by the chief of a major activity. Composite review and analysis is an evaluation of the operation of a department as a whole.

At all levels of management and supervision, some form of appraisal of progress and accomplishment is used. If review and analysis are utilized, they should be a continuous process, with periodic appraisals made at all levels. Generally, review and analysis cycles are divided into four phases: (1) planning; (2) preparation; (3) presentation; and (4) follow-up. Some of these phases may overlap each other if a continuous evaluation program is in progress.

CORRECTING PERFORMANCE

Correction or supplementation of performance implies improvement. Nurse managers should take action to reduce variances with plans by initiating corrective action or supplementation. To initiate corrective action, nurses must (1) understand and accept the responsibility for taking such actions, (2) accept the standards of performance and evaluation as reasonable, necessary, and accurate, (3) be accountable and responsible for correcting discrepancies in their own performance, and (4) regulate and implement the necessary changes.

In taking action to correct or supplement a decision, awareness of the human element involved in the process is critical. Identifying what is wrong is one thing, but getting people to do something about it is quite another matter. People are reluctant to admit deficiencies and they are often resistant to change.

The following guidelines are offered for correcting or improving the performance of nurses in the decision making process.

1. *Set priorities.* Correct the most important discrepancy first. If everything is treated as being equally critical, subordinates will be unable to distinguish what is important from what is routine.

2. *Do not be dogmatic.* By involving subordinates in the decision about what action should be taken to correct the discrepancy, cooperation and support for the action will be strengthened.

3. *Capitalize on the strengths and accomplishments* of the group in correcting discrepancies. Avoid advertising failures of a decision.

4. *Exercise leadership.* Do not permit others to influence your actions too greatly as their perspectives and perceptions may be quite different from yours. Indeed, their perceptions may even be out of line with the realities of the situation.

5. *Be decisive.* It is often better to take an action, even if short of the ideal, than to be indecisive.

6. *Recognize the importance of timing.* Corrective or supplementary action must be

properly timed to take advantage of favorable conditions. The readiness of individuals who will be affected by a decision is also an important dimension of timing.

REFERENCE

1. Bloom, B.: Taxonomy of educational objectives: the classification of educational goals: Handbook I: cognitive domain, New York, 1965, David McKay Co.

SUGGESTED READINGS

Abdellah, F. G., and Levine, E.: Better patient care through nursing research, New York, 1965, The Macmillan Co.

Annas, G. J., and Healey, J.: The patient rights advocate, J. Nurs. Admin. 4:25-31, 1974.

Aradine, C. R., and Pridham, K. F.: Model for collaboration, Nurs. Outlook 21:655-657, 1973.

Aydelotte, M. K.: The use of patient welfare as a criterion measure, Nurs. Res. 11:10-14, 1962.

Bailey, J. T., McDonald, F. J., and Claus, K. E.: An experiment in nursing curriculums at a university, Belmont, Calif., 1972, Wadsworth Publishing Co.

Bidwell, C. M., and Froebe, D. J.: Development of an instrument for evaluating hospital nursing performance, J. Nurs. Admin. 5:10-15, 1971.

Cornell, S. A.: Development of an instrument for measuring the quality of nursing care, Nurs. Res. 23:108-117, 1974.

Cronbach, L. J., and Gleser, G. C.: Psychological tests and personnel decisions, Urbana, 1965, University of Illinois Press.

Ganong, J., Ganong, W., and Huenefeld, J.: Motive force: a key to evaluating nurse managers, J. Nurs. Admin. 4:17-21, 1974.

Gold, H., Jackson, M., Sachs, B., and Van Meter, M. J.: Peer review—a working experiment, Nurs. Outlook 21:634-636, 1973.

Howland, D., and McDowell, W. E.: The measurement of patient care: a conceptual framework, Nurs. Res. 13:4-7, 1964.

Kelly, R. L.: Evaluation is more than measurement, Am. J. Nurs. 73:114-116, 1973.

Mager, R. F.: Measuring instructional intent, Belmont, Calif., 1973, Fearon Publishers.

Pardee, G., Hoshaw, D. O., Huber, C. J., and Larson, B.: Patient care evaluation is every nurses' job, Am. J. Nurs. 71:1958-1960, 1971.

Phaneuf, M. C.: The nursing audit for evaluation of patient care, Nurs. Outlook 14:51-54, 1966.

Popham, W. J., editor: Criterion-referenced measurement, Englewood Cliffs, N. J., 1971, Educational Technology Publications.

Ramphal, M.: Peer review, Am. J. Nurs. 74:63-67, 1974.

Sheps, M.: Approaches to the quality of hospital care, Public Health Reports 70:877-886, 1955.

Waller, M., and Davids, D.: Performance profiles based on nursing activity records, J. Nurs. Admin. 2:60-69, 1972.

Woods, M. F.: Measuring a patient's needs and progress, Nurs. Outlook 60:38-41, 1966.

Zimmer, M. J.: Rationale for a ladder for clinical advancement in nursing practice, J. Nurs. Admin. 2:18-24, 1972.

PART TWO

APPLICATION OF CLAUS-BAILEY MODEL TO NURSING CARE PROBLEMS

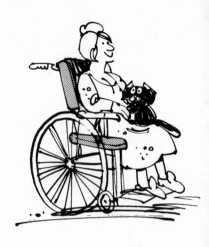

14 THE CLINICAL NURSE SPECIALIST IN A LONG-TERM CARE FACILITY

Relocation of a geriatric patient

SISTER MARY P. QUAYHAGEN, R.N., M.S.

With professional education and clinical expertise, the clinical nurse specialist represents a new role model for leadership and practice. One of the most challenging leadership positions involving direct patient care by nurses is that of the clinical nurse specialist.

At the present time the clinical nurse specialist is generally prepared in advanced educational programs granting masters' degrees. Clinical specialization presupposes in depth knowledge in one specific area and can be linked to age (as with the geriatric clinical specialist), degree of illness (as with the long-term care clinical specialist), body systems (as with the cardiovascular clinical specialist), or clinical services (as with the medical-surgical clinical specialist). These specialists may also function under generalized titles such as the liaison nurse, the home care coordinator, the nursing service coordinator, or the community care coordinator.

In most institutions that provide nursing care to elderly patients, there is an imbalance between the few professionally prepared personnel and the many nonprofessional personnel. The clinician with geriatric expertise is in the position to attempt to bridge this gap through providing patient and staff inservice education and multiagency coordination for patient transfer and discharges. Through inservice education programs, the geriatric clinical specialist can assist members of the nursing staff to gain knowledge and understanding of the aging process, the nursing process as it specifically relates to care of the aging patient, specific pathologies common to the older adult, and the complexities of the decisions facing this patient population.

In addition to the teaching role, the clinical specialist in the geriatric setting will also be able to provide leadership to the health team in demonstrating quality patient care and

---

*From de Beauvoir, S.: The coming of age, New York, 1972, G. P. Putnam's Sons, p. 802.

in planning for patient and family cooperation in the management regimen. By providing greater continuity of care both within the facility and among facilities, the goal of improved delivery of health care services can be achieved.

The geriatric clinical specialist has a role in acute care facilities, long-term facilities, nursing homes, geriatric clinics, and public health or home care agencies. In the following case study, the clinical nurse specialist functioned as a home care coordinator in the long-term care facility.

THE CASE OF THE GERIATRIC PATIENT WITH A PROBLEM OF LIMITED MOBILITY

Mrs. Lillian Low, a 72-year-old widow with no nuclear family, was hospitalized for approximately 4 weeks with a fractured right femur complicated by chronic degenerative arthritis. Mrs. Low reported that she fell on her way home from the store. However, her physician believes that the fracture occurred prior to the fall.

Before the accident, Mrs. Low was living in a second-floor walk-up flat, which she financed with income from her late husband and with social security. She was active in church and community groups, serving as a hospital volunteer 2 days a week and as a foster grandparent to a retarded child 1 day a week. She had been active in her local senior citizens' groups for a number of years. Since she was unable to drive a car, she had been using public transportation for work and social activities. Her apartment was within walking distance of the church and stores.

Mrs. Low's convalescence progressed rapidly following her surgery, which required a total hip replacement. By the fourth week she was transferred from the hospital to the skilled nursing facility for convalescence and rehabilitation. Although Mrs. Low was capable of performing the activities of daily living, her mobility was considerably limited because of the degenerative arthritic changes. She was no longer able to climb stairs or to walk distances.

The home care coordinator for the nursing services at the long-term care facility planned with Mrs. Low for her discharge. Because of the limitations imposed by her physical condition, Mrs. Low had to evaluate her previous life style in terms of her present needs. She had the assistance of the home care coordinator in making the complex decisions inherent in this problem.

In this case study, the home care coordinator who assisted the patient, Mrs. Low, assumed primary responsibility for an easy transition and continuity of care from the long-term care facility to the home situation. The decisions involved in this transition or relocation were complex and called for deliberation of the alternatives. Since the patient did not have access to possible options, the challenge of supplying these options fell to the clinical nurse specialist in her capacity as home care coordinator.

Studies have shown a reluctance among the older persons to become involved in decisions as evidenced by an avoidance of the decision situation. This can be interpreted as a manifestation of much self-doubt and has implications for the clinical setting. Because of the far-reaching consequences, it is essential that the elderly become involved in their discharge planning, which may involve complex decision making. The use of a problem solution model as a tool in the decision making process minimizes the risk involved in relying on subjective judgment and intuition.

DEFINING THE OVERALL NEEDS, PURPOSES, AND GOALS

Define overall needs, purposes, goals

The first step encompassed by the Claus-Bailey Systems Model for Problem Solution is that of defining the overall purposes, needs, and goals.

Purposes. The overall purpose of nursing is the optimal functioning of the patient, physically, psychologically, and socially. A second purpose of nursing, inherent in the first, is to assist the patient toward independent functioning. Both of these purposes are relevant to the problem at hand.

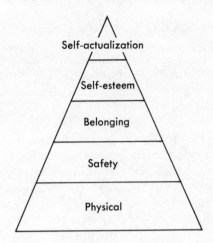

Fig. 14-1. Maslow's theory of motivation.

Needs. In order to more thoroughly assess the overall needs, the Maslow theory of motivation, a positive holistic-dynamic theory, has been selected as the framework.[9] Within this theory the basic human needs are organized into a hierarchy of relative prepotency. In this hierarchy of needs the higher needs are seen to emerge as the lower level needs are gratified. Thus gratification has an important role in Maslow's motivation theory.

The basic needs of man can be differentiated in a hierarchy of five levels (Fig. 14-1). The first level, the physiological, is most basic, encompassing the powerful self-preservation and sexual drives as well as the principles of homeostasis. These needs must generally be met before successive levels of needs assume cognitive import.

Safety and security, the second level of the hierarchy, include the needs for freedom from fear, anxiety, and chaos, as well as the need for protection, stability, and dependency.

On the third level, the belonging or love needs are manifested in the yearnings for affectionate relationships and intimacy. These needs counteract loneliness, alienation, and rejection.

Esteem, the fourth level of the hierarchy, includes the needs for self-respect and a higher evaluation of oneself based on feelings of self-confidence. At this level there is a desire for competence, achievement, recognition, and prestige which fosters self-respect and high self-evaluation.

The top level of the hierarchy, the need for self-actualization, includes self-fulfillment, self-acceptance, and the acceptance of others as exemplified by deep feelings for others expressed through identification and affection. With self-actualization there is a need for simplicity, spontaneity, and creativity. The peak of these needs is the aesthetic or mystic experience, which is independent of culture and environment.

In assessing these needs for a patient, it is necessary to determine the unmet needs. Interventions would then be planned for meeting these needs, beginning with lower level needs and progressing to the higher level needs. In long-term planning and complex decision making, all levels of needs must be viewed simultaneously to determine needs that may arise in the forthcoming situation. Each need may then be assigned a value by the individual, thus aiding in the selection of options.

In evaluating the needs of Mrs. Low, the physiological needs are derived from an understanding of the disease process *per se*. Degenerative arthritis is characterized by a thinning and deterioration of the articular cartilages, by hypertrophy of the bone at the articular margins, and by pain. Older persons are principally affected by the disease, which tends to affect their weight-bearing joints. A decrease in neuromuscular coordination results, as well as mobility limitations. In view of these symptoms, the needs of Mrs. Low are identified as freedom from pain, moderate exercise, sufficient rest, optimal nutrition, and weight control.

The safety and security needs of Mrs. Low are precipitated both by her age and by her disease process, which results in her mobility limitation and her pain. In regard to age, the elderly may be subject to the phenomenon of fear of assault, which must be kept in mind in assessment of the safety and security needs on discharge. These needs for Mrs. Low are thus identified as: (1) security in performing activities of daily living, (2) stability in ambulation demonstrated by the use of available prostheses such as a cane, by the availability of level surfaces without stairs, and by walking only limited distances, (3) protection from vandalism and assault through selection of a relatively crime-free environment if possible, (4) knowledge of the disease process and her prognosis in order to dispel undue fear, and (5) education in self-help modalities necessary for safe ambulation.

The belonging and love needs for Mrs. Low encompass meaningful relationships with friends and associates in church and social activities. The belonging needs also include a familiar neighborhood. The most viable friendships for the elderly often develop within their own peer groups and appear to be enhanced by socioeconomic equality.

Variables that give impetus to esteem needs for Mrs. Low are those of her previous role interaction and her previous high level of independence, both of which will be somewhat changed by disease limitations. Another variable is that of an altered body image and self-concept caused by the chronicity role she must now assume. Therefore esteem needs may be enumerated as: (1) continuation of meaningful rewarding activities such as her volunteer and foster grandparent work and senior citizen activity, (2) perception of self as independent and competent, (3) positive feedback from peer relations, and (4) environment in which independent mastery is a reality.

Self-actualization needs are difficult to identify from a case study. However, for Mrs. Low these needs appear to be those of self-acceptance in the face of her imposed limitations and a continuation of energy investment in outer objects. The variables of altered body image, social limitations, and physical restrictions influence these needs.

Goals. The goals for Mrs. Low are the following.

1. To attain independent physical functioning as measured by ability to perform without assistance the activities of daily living, as well as the management of her own living environment
2. To procure a safe environment with personal security as evidenced by the presence of hand rails in areas of unsure footing and where major positional changes are required, e.g., the bathroom; by the absence of assault on her person or possessions; and by freedom from fear caused by inadequate knowledge of her disease process or prognosis
3. To sustain meaningful relationships as evidenced by frequent visits with a peer in whom she can confide and by association with church group and social group
4. To find rewarding social involvement as measured by self report of feelings of satisfaction in volunteer activities, and by verbal awareness of herself as independent and competent
5. To attain self-acceptance as evidenced by ability to admit imposed limitations and to continue to invest her energy in external objects and persons

The discrepancy

After thoroughly assessing the overall needs, it is necessary to identify the discrepancy which is an obstacle to the attainment of the needs at the various levels. In reviewing the five levels of needs it can be noticed that the physiological and safety needs have been altered by her pathological state, while the love, esteem, and self-actualization needs remain the same for Mrs. Low as in the prepathological state. The disease process has resulted in this alteration. Comparing Mrs. Low's physical abilities prior to her fall with those of her present condition, it becomes apparent that the discrepancy rests in her present living situation— the second floor walk-up apartment with its stairs and distances.

THE PROBLEM

Define problem

In analyzing the above discrepancy, it can be seen that the problem of Mrs. Low is her mobility limitations resulting in the necessity to relocate into housing that allows for maximum mobility. A new housing situation cannot have stairs and must be within shorter walking distances of church and stores. Since the discrepancy is limited to the physical structure of the building itself, a similar socioeconomic neighborhood or the same neighborhood should be chosen as the site of the new location. The problem actually began when Mrs. Low fell; with the treatment of the fracture, the degenerative arthritic condition was discovered. The extent of the problem is limited to her ambulatory restrictions, which necessitate the relocation.

Studies of relocation and the elderly have primarily focused on relocation into an institution or between institutions.[1,3,10,11] Some of the findings from these studies have implications for the elderly person relocating in the community. Markus and associates conceptualize relocation as consisting of two stages, one in which the person is deprived of his usual environmental supports and familiar cues, and the second in which the person must adjust to new stimuli in an unfamiliar environment.[8] In adjusting to the new environment the impact of relocation may be lessened if there is congruency between the personality of the individual and the adaptive demands of the environment. A style of active participation and interaction seems well fitted to relocation as a combatant of isolation. Relocation can be seen as a problem in light of the high mortality and morbidity rates, which may be attributed to maladjustment. High postrelocation mortality rate has been documented and occurs most frequently within the first year, often within the first 3 months after relocation. Therefore, when faced with the decision of relocation, the individual must seriously consider all available alternatives in the light of his previous lifestyle and environment and present coping abilities.

CONSTRAINTS AND RESOURCES

Specify constraints, capabilities, resources, claimant groups

The constraints and capabilities or resources can be identified through force field analysis.[5] These can be viewed as positive and negative forces impinging upon the situation. The constraints are then visualized as the resisting forces, while the capabilities and resources become the pushing forces. Each of these forces and the ratio of their relative strengths are presented in Fig. 14-2. The percentage or ratio of strength is that perceived by the patient with validation of the nurse. As can be seen from Fig. 14-2, Mrs. Low's chief constraint is that of mobility restrictions, while her major capabilities or resources are the ability to control her pain, her close peer group relationships, and her positive self-concept.

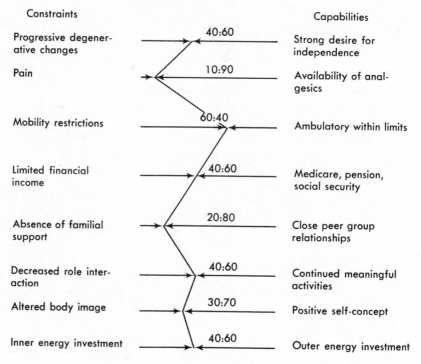

Fig. 14-2. Analysis of resisting and pushing forces.

THE APPROACH

Specify approach to problem solution

If a single, all-encompassing theoretical approach is desirable here, it is that of the activity theory of successful aging in which the philosophical belief is that life satisfaction is contingent upon continuity of the activity patterns of middle life into later life. Freedom of choice and independence are strongly implicit in this theory.

Inherent in this approach are ten basic assumptions.[2,6,7]

1. That independence in physiological and psychosocial functioning is a desirable goal for man, regardless of age

2. That progressive degenerative changes associated with chronic disabilities in the elderly will result in progressive mobility limitations

3. That a physically safe and socially secure environment is essential for optimal functioning

4. That peer confidante relationships are essential for life satisfaction of elderly persons without close familial ties

5. That continued interpersonal contacts and involvements will be necessary for life satisfaction of elderly patients who were previously involved

6. That freedom of choice is the basic human right of people in a democracy

7. That man is a rational being who, when confronted with a decision situation, will select the optimal choice

8. That despite the aging process, man retains the ability to solve problems and make decisions

9. That the nurse, theoretically prepared in leadership and decision making skills, has the potential and responsibility for assisting the patient in decision deliberations that have implications for health delivery

10. That the capability of the elderly to optimally meet lower level needs is a prerequisite to life satisfaction and self-fulfillment

Therefore the theoretical approach is that of continuing involvement as encompassed by the activity theory of successful aging, with freedom of choice and independence.

BEHAVIORAL OBJECTIVES AND PERFORMANCE CRITERIA

State behavioral objectives and performance criteria

The specific behavioral objective for Mrs. Low is for her to select freely, with the consultation of the clinical nurse specialist, the optimal physical and psychosocial living situation allowing for minimal alterations of previous life style.

The performance criteria include the attainment of independent physical and psychosocial functioning for Mrs. Low, as well as management of her own living situation. In addition, there must be a safe environment as measured by her freedom from falls and other hazards to health, by her freedom from undue fears, and by absence of assault to her person or property.

Her close confidante relationships can be measured by the frequency of her visits and by verbal reports of the quality of these interactions. Also, in the new situation, the ability to find a new confidante will in itself be a measure of this objective.

Mrs. Low's attendance at church and other social functions and her active participation in the interaction are criteria for measuring this objective.

That Mrs. Low reestablishes a positive self-concept can be determined by her verbal reports of acceptance of her changed image in view of her now present disability.

Last, the utilization of opportunities for creative thought and action by Mrs. Low will be determined by her mental and/or physical productivity, which might be abstract and very difficult to measure.

ALTERNATIVE SOLUTIONS

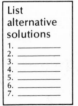

List alternative solutions
1. _____
2. _____
3. _____
4. _____
5. _____
6. _____
7. _____

The role of the home care coordinator in assisting the patient with her decision is to locate all possible alternatives of living situations, in view of Mrs. Low's present limitations necessitating her relocation. Since one of her belonging needs is identified as the need for a familiar neighborhood, the search should logically begin in the immediate environment of her present apartment. However, there are no structures or facilities without stairs in Mrs. Low's neighborhood. Therefore the search was extended to comparable socioeconomic neighborhoods and revealed the following six alternatives:

1. A retirement home with elevator and available health care clinic, patterned on the lifetime care concept. The patient lives in the retirement section until such time as she needs care, and then is placed in the nursing unit.

2. An apartment (in a building with an elevator) which is located near a clinic or health maintenance organization.

3. A retirement hotel near the same clinic or health maintenance organization. The retirement hotel provides for independent living, with meals available in three dining areas. However, once the patient can no longer maintain herself, a further move will be necessary, for no nursing care is available there.

4. A ground-level house, also near the clinic or health maintenance organization, that can be rented for a nominal fee.

5. A mobile home retirement community with ramp and available health follow-up facilities. The mobile home community does not have lifetime care available, but does have a transfer agreement with a local nursing home facility should such care be necessary. The follow-up facilities consist of a clinic that operates 5 days a week in the mobile home court.

6. A skilled nursing facility, which is also a home for aged patients, giving them lifetime care.

ANALYSIS OF OPTIONS

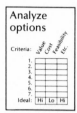

In analyzing the options or alternatives, it is necessary to establish specific criteria against which these options will be measured. The criteria for analyzing the alternatives available to Mrs. Low are determined from the needs that appear in the assessment according to the hierarchy of needs, and are inherent in the behavioral objectives and performance criteria. These criteria include: (1) availability of health care, (2) number of stairs, (3) walking distances, (4) private transportation (since she cannot climb the steps on the public transit vehicles), (5) financial cost, (6) personal safety, (7) risk of change, (8) available confidante (from previously established contact), (9) peer group contacts, (10) peer activities, (11) amount of independence, and (12) overall value to the patient. An analysis of these options is presented in Fig. 14-3. A scoring range of "Hi," "Mod," and "Lo" is used to designate high, moderate, or low desirability for each criterion measure. The ideal score for each is also established.

It can be seen from Fig. 14-3 that Option 1, the retirement home with the elevator and lifetime care concept, most closely meets the ideal. The mobile home retirement community is only one point behind the retirement home. Hoever, it is at this point that the decision rules must be discussed and applied.

DECISION RULES

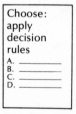

The first of the decision rules is that the patient, when confronted with the decision situation, will select the option that has the greatest value and the lowest risk. In looking at Fig. 14-3 and Options 1 and 5, and applying this decision rule to them, it can be noticed that they are both of moderate risk since they are outside the familiar neighborhood but are in a neighborhood that is similar to the patient's present environment. They also have high overall value to Mrs. Low for the same reason. Therefore, this decision rule is inconclusive here.

The second decision rule is to select that option which is financially feasible. This rule thus becomes the discriminating rule in the case of Mrs. Low, as the retirement home with the lifetime care concept is very costly and therefore not financially feasible to her. The opposite is true of the mobile home community, as it is relatively low in cost and is financially feasible.

The third decision is to select from the financially feasible choices that one which provides for physical independence and optimal psychosocial involvement. It is not necessary to apply this rule since only one of the two top options is financially feasible.

Ideal	Options						Criteria
	1	2	3	4	5	6	
Hi	(Hi)	Mod	Mod	Mod	(Hi)	(Hi)	Availability of health care
Lo	(Lo)	(Lo)	(Lo)	(Lo)	(Lo)	(Lo)	Number of stairs
Lo	(Lo)	Mod	Mod	Mod	Mod	(Lo)	Walking distances
Hi	(Hi)	Lo	Mod	Lo	(Hi)	(Hi)	Private transportation
Lo	Hi	Mod	Hi	Mod	(Lo)	Hi	Financial cost
Hi	(Hi)	Lo	(Hi)	Mod	Mod	(Hi)	Personal safety
Lo	Mod	Hi	Mod	Hi	Mod	Hi	Risk of change
Hi	Lo	Lo	Lo	Lo	Lo	Lo	Available confidante
Hi	(Hi)	Lo	(Hi)	Lo	(Hi)	Mod	Peer group contacts
Hi	(Hi)	Lo	Mod	Lo	(Hi)	(Hi)	Peer activities
Hi	(Hi)	(Hi)	(Hi)	(Hi)	(Hi)	Lo	Amount of independence
Hi	(Hi)	Mod	(Hi)	Mod	(Hi)	Lo	Overall value to patient
	9	2	5	2	8	6	Score

Fig. 14-3. Analysis of the options.

IMPLEMENTATION

Control
and
implement
decisions

Following the application of the decision rules, Mrs. Low chose the fifth alternative, the mobile home retirement community with the available health care clinic. To assist Mrs. Low in implementing the decision, the nursing home care coordinator took the following actions: (1) arranged with the management of the retirement community to have someone assist Mrs. Low to select a suitable available mobile home and to move her belongings, (2) visited the mobile home to ascertain if safety features were adequate and maximum independence possible, (3) arranged for referral of Mrs. Low's health history and records to the follow-up health care clinic, and (4) emotionally supported Mrs. Low as she disengaged psychologically from her previous location and friends and reengaged or reinvested her energy in her new environment.

Once the decision was made, reinforcement and reassurance were necessary. Contacts were made in advance of her arrival to the senior citizens' group in the retirement community so that a welcome was planned for her. This facilitated her establishing new friendships.

EVALUATION

Evaluate effectiveness of action

The effectiveness of Mrs. Low's relocation into the mobile home retirement community was substantiated by her adjustment to the new location. An evaluation of this effectiveness was determined by application of the previously established criteria as identified under goals and performance criteria for the behavioral objectives.

In regard to independence in physiological and psychosocial functioning, Mrs. Low was able to perform all the activities of daily living and to manage the housekeeping of her mobile home without assistance. However, because of the continued degeneration physically, she can anticipate that in a few years she will be transferred to the skilled nursing facility.

In regard to the physically safe and socially secure environment, Mrs. Low has not had any recurring falls nor has she encountered any additional hazards in her mobile home. She has had safety rails placed in the bathroom facilities and has lowered the closet racks to eliminate unnecessary and hazardous reaching. The ramp outside already had a guard rail. The mobile home community has a security patrol for the protection of the residents from assault or robbery. Therefore Mrs. Low's environment is physically safe and secure.

Mrs. Low has continued her medical follow-up and is presently relatively free from pain with her continued use of a prescribed analgesic. The clinic has transportation for her to and from her mobile home.

Mrs. Low has made many friends from her participation in the church and social activities in the mobile home community, but she has not yet established a confidante peer relationship to replace her previous relationship. Because of this, she has expressed a feeling of loneliness which she did not have in her former situation. She has continued and is continuing her other social activities except for the foster grandparent and volunteer work. She verbalized her disappointment at not being able to continue these functions.

Mrs. Low has verbalized that it has been harder to accept herself with her limitations than she had anticipated. She believed that her previous abilities would slowly return, but has now been faced with the reality that further limitations will be forthcoming. However, she has continued to invest her energy in objects and persons outside herself and has expressed a desire to keep active as long as possible.

As part of her rehabilitation therapy, Mrs. Low has become interested in clay modeling. This has also provided a creative outlet for her.

Thus it can be seen from the evaluation based on the established criteria that Mrs. Low's decision to relocate in the mobile home community was basically effective.

SUMMARY

The effectiveness of the use of the Claus-Bailey Systems Model for Problem Solution has been demonstrated in its application to the complex problem of relocation which faces many of the elderly today. When an elderly person is a patient in a long-term care facility, a nurse is often delegated the role of assisting the patient in the decision making process. Thus effective leadership and decision making skills are essential to patient-centered care as nursing becomes more autonomous and professional.

REFERENCES

1. Aldrich, C., and Mendkoff, E.: Relocation of the aged and disabled: A mortality study, J. Am. Geriatr. Soc. **11:**185-194, 1963.
2. Beeson, P. B., and McDermott, W.: Cecil-Loeb textbook of medicine, ed. 13, Philadelphia, 1971, W. B. Saunders Co.
3. Blenkner, M.: Environmental change and the aging individual, Gerontologist **7:**101-105, 1967.
4. de Beauvoir, S.: The coming of age, New York, 1972, G. P. Putnam's Sons.
5. Lewin, K.: Field theory in social science, New York, 1951, Harper & Row, Publishers.
6. Lowenthal, M. F., and Haven, C.: Interaction and adaptation intimacy as a critical variable, Am. Sociol. Rev. **33:**20-30, 1968.
7. Maddox, G., and Eisdorfer, C.: Some correlates of activity and morale among the elderly, Social Forces **40:**354-260, 1962.
8. Markus, E., and others: Some factors and their association with post-relocation mortality among institutionalized aged persons, J. Gerontol. **27:**376-382, 1972.
9. Maslow, A. H.: Motivation and personality, ed. 2, New York, 1970, Harper & Row, Publishers.
10. Miller, D., and Lieberman, M. A.: The relationship of affect state and adaptive capacity to reactions to stress, J. Gerontol. **20:**492-497, 1965.
11. Turner, B. F., Tobin, S. S., and Lieberman, M. A.: Personality traits as predictors of institutional adaption among the aged, J. Gerontol. **27:**61-68, 1972.

SUGGESTED READINGS

Anderson, H. C.: Newton's geriatric nursing, ed. 2, St. Louis, 1971, The C. V. Mosby Co.
Botwinick, J.: Aging and behavior, New York, 1973, Springer Publishing Co.
Brody, S. J.: Comprehensive health care for the elderly: An analysis, Gerontologist **13:**412-418, 1973.
Carp, F. M.: A future for the aged, Austin, 1966, University of Texas.
Georgopoulos, B. S., and Christman, L.: The clinical nurse specialist: A role model, The Clinical Nurse Specialist, New York, 1970, American Journal of Nursing Co.
Lee, W.: Decision theory and human behavior, New York, 1971, John Wiley & Sons, Inc.
Rosow, I.: Social integration of the aged, New York, 1967, The Free Press.

The true measure of the value of nursing service rests in the
degree to which it modifies the health behavior of others.

R. B. FREEMAN*

15 A NURSING SERVICE DIRECTOR IN AN ACUTE HEALTH CARE CENTER

Quality control of nursing care

EARLINE L. BRYAN, R.N., M.S.

Today we are in the midst of change. Increasing technology and the concept of health as a basic human right have created new and extended roles for health professionals. There is an increased emphasis upon health maintenance and preventive services that will move many of the nursing services out of institutional settings and into diverse settings within the total community.

The director of nursing service will be responsible for a group of people who must interdependently relate to a large, continually growing, and extremely complex array of health care personnel. The director's scope of responsibility will be: (1) to facilitate quality care through the provision of equipment, materials, and educational resources, (2) to direct others, (3) to communicate policy decisions and procedural changes, (4) to provide a work environment that promotes patient and employee well-being, (5) to maintain a well-qualified staff through selection procedures and to provide professional development, (6) to assist others in developing both personal and professional goals, which can be evaluated, (7) to support the research process through conducting studies, implementing and sharing the findings, and (8) to coordinate and integrate services within the agency and among agencies for the enhancement of patient care.[11]

The challenge presented to nursing directors, then, is to bring about change within the systems as health services evolve from management of acute illness to the prevention of illness and to health maintenance. Nursing service must redirect its focus from a task-oriented base to a patient-centered approach.

Methods for establishing accountability, standards of care, quality control, and efficiency measurements must be incorporated in the plan for the delivery of nursing care

---

*From Freeman, R. B.: Techniques of supervision in public health nursing, ed. 2, Philadelphia, 1949, W. B. Sanders Co.

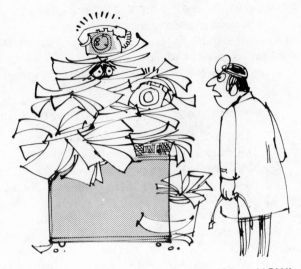

Fig. 15-1. I need the records for Mrs. Green NOW!

and rehabilitative functions. A system of delivery of nursing service designed to improve quality of nursing care that includes the development of standards, surveillance, and corrective action is one approach directed toward meeting patient needs.

Obviously the director of nursing bears the ultimate responsibility for the department's quality control program, as well as for other aspects of nursing care services. Developing standards of performance is one of the most critical needs in the delivery of health care. Standards of performance need to be made explicit and upheld by both nursing management and nurses who provide the care. The director of nursing should work with all levels of nurses to develop standards of performance. Although the director must depend on various nursing staff members to formulate specific standards and patient care objectives, the director should have some general standards in mind that are clearly focused on excellence and on quality patient care. Thus the director can promote a viable quality control program by first developing standards of performance that can be used as criteria in the development of a quality control program. The development and effectiveness of such a program becomes essentially the responsibility of the nursing service director.

REQUISITES TO THE IMPLEMENTATION OF A QUALITY CONTROL SYSTEM IN AN ACUTE HEALTH CARE CENTER

Selection, implementation, and evaluation of a quality control system require skills in the problem solving and decision making processes. Approaches and alternatives must be planned, generated, and evaluated. Since members of nursing service look to nursing service directors for leadership as they deal with problems, directors need to have a variety of tools and techniques to assist them in their leadership role. The Claus-Bailey Systems Model for Problem Solution is one such technique that enables a director of nursing service and the nursing staff to become involved in solving complex problems of quality control.

The focus of this chapter is to demonstrate the use of the Claus-Bailey Model as a tool in selecting, implementing, and evaluating a quality control system from the perspective of a director of nursing service in an acute care center. This approach exposes basic problems, assists with the measurement of critical variables, and aids in the prediction of the consequences of various alternatives. The use of such a model minimizes the risk involved when one relies solely on subjective judgement and intuition in the decision making process.

DEFINING THE OVERALL NEEDS, PURPOSES, AND GOALS

The first step in this problem solving approach is that of defining the overall purposes, needs, and goals.

Purposes. The primary purposes of a quality control system in a health care institution are to identify deficiencies in patient care and to improve the quality of patient care. Subpurposes are related to supervision of the patient and of those participating in the care, and to effecting changes in performance and improving practice through a detached, critical inquiry into quality.

Needs. The overall properties and needs of a viable quality control system are standards, surveillance, and corrective action. Standards refer to that which can be observed and measured. Standards for nursing care fall into two groups: the nursing practices (the process of care) and the outcome of the care. Standards of care derive from research, expert group judgment, and observation of the way nursing and medicine are actually practiced. Standards must be developed before nursing care can be evaluated. Once standards have been developed they require periodic review and revision.

Surveillance consists of comparing the care given with the standards expected. This entails an anlysis of data derived from the review of the care given based on a chart review of direct evaluation of the patient in the care setting.

The feedback loop presented in Fig. 3-1 is a mechanism for guiding corrective action that must be taken when discrepancies are noted between performance and standards. Such actions may include education, recommendations related to changes in present practice, and intervention such as withdrawal of privileges for those who do not provide care that meets established standards. Additionally, scheduled progress (timetables) toward the achievement of the standards is crucial if quality control is to become a reality, not merely a theory.

Goals. The goals for a quality control system are the following:

1. To ensure a system that will optimize quality effectivenes and performance as measured by a comparison of the care provided with measurable, predetermined standards
2. To plan and coordinate an audit program that will result in increased effectiveness and improved patient care by identifying deficiencies so that changes in performance of practice can be effected
3. To take effective corrective actions when problems are found in the patient care processes to assure nonreoccurrence, by improving performance through inservice education directed toward improved patient care

The discrepancy

Following the assessment of needs and the determination of the purpose and specific objectives, it is essential that the discrepancy be identified so that obstacles to needs and goal fulfillment can be eliminated. In reviewing the needs it can be ascertained that obstacles to the determination of quality care relate to a lack of measurable standards of care, continuous surveillance through an audit, and a lack of prompt corrective action to rectify existent discrepancies. Additionally, the literature is replete with instances of inaccurate, incomplete, subjective documentation of care in the clinical record—an obstacle to the evaluation of the quality of patient care.

THE PROBLEM

Define
problem

The first requirement before moving to decision making is to determine if the problem is clearly defined and fully understood. If the problem is not defined and understood, it cannot be solved properly. From the discrepancy described above, it can be noted that the problem has been defined as the necessity to develop standards for measuring the quality of patient care provided by health professionals.

Studies relating to the evaluation of quality care have primarily focused on structure, process, or outcomes using a variety of sources for quality control checks: charts, rounds, records, nursing care plans, patient interviews, nurse interviews, and interviews of other health personnel. Each is useful for the specific purpose for which it was designed; each has its limitations as a measure of quality of care.[4,10,17-19]

Medical practice and nursing practice in hospitals are often selected as subjects of study for both practical and theoretical reasons. A frequent assumption is that there is a relationship between quality of medical and nursing practices within hospitals and within the community at large. Furthermore, intensive community organization of health service is generally focused on organized facilities. In addition, hospital service constitutes an important segment of medical and nursing care in the community. Finally, the hospital is an organized medical care facility that provides a practical focus for study. Because evaluation of a sufficient number of cases by direct observation would be costly, medical records are often used as the basis for evaluation.

Studies have shown that, in addition to limitations in reliability of clinical evaluation, other serious limitations are imposed by generally deficient records. This deficiency has implications for a need for restudy of the form and content of the medical record. Therefore, when faced with the decision of implementing a quality control system, the designated committee in conjunction with the nursing director must consider all available alternatives with respect to cost, feasibility of implementation, availability of a logical system, reliability, and simplicity for use.

CONSTRAINTS AND CAPABILITIES

Specify
constraints,
capabilities,
resources,
claimant
groups

The constraints and capabilties or resources can best be determined through a force field analysis.[8] These can be visualized as forces that initiate a change and keep it going (driving forces or capabilities) and forces that retard movement toward a goal (restraining forces or constraints). The force field is made up of forces of varying strengths that oppose each other. The ratios of the relative strengths are depicted in Fig. 15-2. The ration of strength is that perceived by the individual doing the analysis. From Fig. 15-2, it becomes apparent that the major capabilities are financial support, staff and administrative interest in assessing and improving patient care, and availability of assessment criteria for evaluation of patient care. The chief constraint relates to strict adherence to rules.

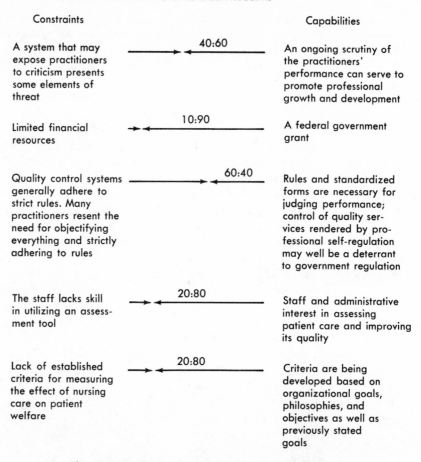

Fig. 15-2. Analysis of restraining and pushing forces.

THE APPROACH

Specify approach to problem solution

In any effort to improve the care of patients, definitive standards for practice must be clearly established. Likewise generally deficient clinical records pose serious limitations to evaluation of patient care based on the study of medical records. Inherent in this approach are the following assumptions.

1. The ideal method of quality measurement is one that assures the same evaluation in any given case when the method is applied by independent observers.

2. The patient care record (an instrument of services rendered) is one important basis for quality appraisal.

3. The effectiveness of a team approach to comprehensive patient care is contingent on an accurate, efficient record.

4. Nursing will continue to be based upon empirical, intuitive approaches until such time that nurses begin to maintain permanent records of the effects of their interventions in specific patient care problems.

5. Professional nurses should be responsible for appraising nursing practice and service.

6. Professional groups with varying responsibilities for patient care must interface in a systematic and collaborative fashion.

7. Nurses can detect nursing service deficiencies and other related aspects of care by direct inspection of patients, their environment, and their medical records. Nurses can compare the data collected with predetermined standards for nursing care and services.[1-3,9,12,17]

Therefore the approach will be that of reorganization of the medical record to allow for evaluation of patient care; development of standards and objective criteria by a committee of experts; conduct of a pre-audit to determine the present level of care which will serve as a baseline for future comparison; and an analysis of incidents of effective and ineffective nursing care to note differences in quality.

BEHAVIORAL OBJECTIVES

State behavioral objectives and performance criteria

The behavioral objectives include the following.

1. To revise the organization of medical records to allow for a meaningful audit in the practice of nursing and medicine
2. To provide measures that will indicate the level of the quality of care and services—the degree of nursing proficiency
3. To provide such measures on a continuing basis as a vital ongoing management control
4. To provide feedback in order to allow the necessary corrective action

PERFORMANCE CRITERIA

The following performance criteria were developed to assess the extent to which the system is functioning.

1. Medical records will conform to accepted and predetermined standards.
2. The system will be operative, logical, and understood by members who are using it.
3. Improvement in patient care by a predetermined timetable will be documented.
4. Documentation will describe how well the delivery of patient care measures up to standards.
5. Written standards of quality of the care will be provided.
6. Written recommendations to management regarding corrective action with regard to discrepancies will be available.
7. Written evidence of the enforcement of quality control will be available.
8. Records of changes in practice will be noted.
9. Evidence will be available to confirm that educational programs take place when discrepancies are noted between performance and standards.

ALTERNATIVE SOLUTIONS

List alternative solutions
1. _____
2. _____
3. _____
4. _____
5. _____
6. _____
7. _____

The next step involves assessing all possible alternatives of quality control systems. Obtaining as much factual information as possible is critical. The facts must be examined and challenged prior to deciding on a course of action. This approach will assist the staff in identifying the methods that could be used along with their comparative advantages and disadvantages. The previous examination step will have provided many new and different ideas and suggestions. The next step is to select the best possible solution from among them, and one likely to produce the best results.

Discussions and research by a task force resulted in the generation of four plausible alternatives:

1. Problem-Oriented Medical Records (POMR) supplemented by standards of care
2. Nursing audit
3. Task-analysis method
4. Peer review

A brief summary of each of the alternative solutions will be presented before discussing the next step in the problem solution process.

The problem-oriented medical record (POMR). The problem-oriented medical record evaluates the critical thinking of the practitioner by allowing an audit of the record to determine what care was given and the logic behind each intervention. Properly utilized, the POMR provides a logical, precise list of all the patient's problems, current treatment, and plans of the health team relative to each problem. A chart review is an efficient means of evaluating the team's performance and provides the practitioner with instant, meaningful feedback on the quality of patient care. The problem-oriented record does not allow the user to separate the process and outcome, or allow one problem to be considered out of the context with other problems. Therefore both the process and the outcome are jointly evaluated. The problem-oriented system of record keeping, relative to patient management, may provide a common approach for nursing, medicine, and other health professionals. This mutual orientation should enhance collaborative attempts toward defining and developing congruent roles. Since the problem-oriented record outlines problems and assigns names to them, it can serve as a source of statistical data in reviewing patient care from records. Likewise, problems can be categorized and used to study the care given by interdisciplinary health care personnel. This type of record promotes continuity of care by allowing any health professional to review the problems, plans, treatment, and follow-up on a selected patient. The problem-oriented medical record is also a system for quality control at a fairly reasonable cost.

The nursing audit. The nursing audit is based on a process approach to evaluation, and seems to answer the question, "Does the patient receive good nursing care?" The descriptive statements related to the components under each of the seven nursing functions do not focus on the outcome of care, but rather on the process. Therefore no attempt is made to evaluate the outcome of care.

The nursing audit lacks the basis for professional collaboration since it evaluates only nursing care. Joint assessment of quality care by members of the health care team appears to be requisite if the total quality of patient care is to be determined.

The nursing audit does evaluate the critical thinking of the nurse practitioners in relation to their ability to interrelate past and present illness, knowledge of disease, expected therapeutic results, and untoward side effects, and has been described as a tool that enables one to obtain a detached inquiry into measurement of quality.

Information obtained from the nursing audit may lend itself to the study of nursing in a systematic manner; however, the basis of the development of the nursing audit was not a research operation. Comparative studies between agencies, using a standardized form, are needed to establish reliability and validity of the instrument.

Task-analysis method. The task-analysis method is a system developed to distribute nursing tasks in a fair manner. The basic criterion measure focuses on what is being done rather than what should be done. The system perceives nursing as a series of specific tasks, and is oriented toward what happens in the care delivery system rather than what happens to the patient. The method assigns point values to selected nursing tasks and selected patient states. Each point value is converted into an estimated number of hours of nursing care. While this system is useful in patient care and staff placement, it appears that the system is unable to function as a quality control system.[15,18]

Peer review. Peer review is oriented toward the manageability of the nursing role rather than toward the management of nursing care problems. Presently its criteria do not focus on nursing process and patient outcomes. Group cohesiveness is often reduced as practitioners are reluctant to judge and be judged. Many nurses feel threatened by a peer review process. Lack of established criteria as a baseline for evaluation precludes the conduct of an objective peer review. Once criteria have been developed, peer review may become an accepted means to examine and evaluate practice. Additionally, it may serve as a measure of accountability and as a means of evaluating and improving standards of practice.

ANALYSIS OF OPTIONS

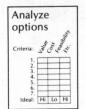

An analysis of the options or alternatives requires a comparison of the alternatives against specific, measurable criteria. The criteria for analyzing the alternatives available to the staff were determined from the needs that are inherent in a quality control system, and those stated in the behavioral objectives and performance criteria. These criteria include: (1) feasibility of implementation, (2) financial cost, (3) risk of change— threat to practitioner, (4) reliable indicator of quality, (5) provision for corrective action and surveillance, (6) applicability to several specialties and general wards, (7) time, (8) provision for accurate recording of objective observations in the clinical record, (9) retrievability of data from the record, (10) availability of measurable standards of performance, and (11) overall value to patient care. An analysis of these options appear in Fig. 15-3. The range of scoring of "Hi," "Mod," and Lo" designates high, moderate, or low value for each criterion measure. The ideal score for each criterion is also designated.

As noted in Fig. 15-3, Option 1, implementation of problem-oriented medical records (POMR) and the development of measurable standards for evaluation, most closely measures up to the ideal. The nursing audit lagged three points behind the POMR. Thus we must proceed to a discussion and application of the decision rules.

DECISION RULES

Three major decision rules can serve as guidelines in the decision sequence.

1. When dealing with problems of patient care, high-risk procedures should generally be avoided. The objective is to promote a viable system which will provide precise data to be utilized as a diagnostic tool in bringing about quality and comprehensive patient care.

2. The second decision rule involves cost, which should be within the budget allocation and also meet the objective—quality patient care.

3. As an instrument of care evaluation the method of measurement should be: (a) "sufficiently sensitive to distinguish differences in the quality of care among units being evaluated; (b) objective in that different observers would arrive at similar ranking of units with similar magnitudes of differences between them; (c) valid in that it would reflect the quality of service in terms of current concepts of good medical and nursing practice; (d) based on sufficiently general principles of medical and nursing practice to the appli-

Ideal	Options				Criteria
	1	2	3	4	
Hi	(Hi)	(Hi)	Mod	(Hi)	Feasibility of implementation
Lo	Mod+	Mod	Hi	(Lo)	Financial cost
Lo	Mod	Mod	(Lo)	Mod	Risk of change—threat to practitioner
Hi	(Hi)	Mod	Lo	Lo	Reliable indicator of quality
Hi	(Hi)	(Hi)	Lo	Mod	Permits corrective action and surveillance
Hi	(Hi)	(Hi)	(Hi)	(Hi)	Applicable to several specialties and general ward use
Short	Mod to Long	Mod	Mod	Mod	Time to implement
Hi	(Hi)	Lo	Lo	Lo	Permits accurate recording of objective observations in record
Hi	(Hi)	Mod	Lo	Lo	Retrievable data from record
Hi	(Hi)	(Hi)	Mod	Lo	Availability of measurable standards of care and performance
Hi	(Hi)	(Hi)	Mod	Lo	Overall value to patient care
	8	5	2	3	Score

Fig. 15-3. Analysis of the options.

cable to several specialties; (e) practical of application at costs that are not prohibitive," and (f) flexible enough to permit joint assessment of total patient care by members of several professions.[13,17]

In comparing Options 1 and 2 (presented in Fig. 15-3) and in applying the first decision rule, it can be noted that they are both of moderate risk since they subject the practitioner's performance to scrutiny. However, detection of discrepancies in performance followed by corrective action enhances the quality of care. Therefore Option 1, which permits accurate data to be retrieved from the record for an audit, is better.

The second decision rule relates to the cost of implementation. Instituting the problem-oriented medical record (POMR) is initially more costly than the nursing audit. However, the POMR appears to have greater value as a detector of quality care since it provides a disciplined format to be followed which can lead to improved care. Additionally, a grant is available to cover costs of implementation and continuance of the system. Thus Option 1 is the ideal system.

Application of the third decision rule to Options 1 and 2 reveals a discrepancy in the auditing method of Option 2. The nursing audit lacks the basis for professional collaboration since it separately evaluates nursing care. Joint assessment by members of several professions is required for evaluation of total patient care. The POMR has this capability since all professionals who provide patient care and service document their contributions in one progress note. Therefore Option 1 is the ideal choice.

Gain acceptance. The important action here is communication. Adequate communication is critical at this stage. Everyone needs to be informed of the final decision and concerted efforts made to gain acceptance and approval. Once acceptance is achieved, the proposed solution can be implemented.

IMPLEMENTATION

Following the application of the decision rules, the nursing director and the quality control committee choose the first alternative—the problem-oriented medical record (POMR) supplemented by standards of care and performance. To assist the staff in implementing the decision, the nursing director, coordinator, consultant, and inservice educator take the following actions: (1) collaborate with a committee of experts in developing standards of quality care, (2) arrange for the conduct of a pre-audit (by the audit committee) to assess the present level of care, (3) designate a committee to take corrective action when discrepancies are noted in performance, (4) collaborate with a committee to develop a standardized data base form so that a basic amount of territory is convered, (5) collaborate with the staff in writing protocols for frequently occurring disease entities using the SOAP (subjective, objective, assessment, and plan) format and devising the necessary flow sheets, (6) designate the medical care unit as the unit that makes the transition to the problem-oriented system as an exercise in planned change,* (7) inform the staff that the coordinator, inservice educator, the consultant will assist with practice in charting in the SOAP format and will audit patients' charts at specified intervals—helping individual nurses as needed (a physician from the medical records department can also audit the physician's entries), (8) determine that the system is instituted with the arrival of new residents and interns who are familiar with this system, (9) set a timetable for the achievement of standards and evaluation of the viability of the POMR system (setting time limits on goals helps to see results), (10) publicize that this form of charting should begin on the nurses' notes and eventually progress to entries on a single progress note, (11) make plans for eventual adaptation of nursing care plans to problem lists, (12) inform the staff that data base forms will be revised periodically to perfect the system, (13) designate the physician as the formulator of the patient problem list, and (14) establish change relationships with the staff as they make the transition from source-oriented records to problem-oriented records.

Prior to the implementation of the problem-oriented record system members of the staff should begin to familiarize themselves with the use of the system through reading related literature, viewing films on the subject, and meeting with a nurse consultant. These meetings should occur twice a month and establish the climate for change, which facilitates a smoother transition to POMR.

> Control and implement decisions

---

*Other units can attempt to make this change at a later time. Since reports indicate that adaptation to the POMR system occurs more quickly in specialty units and since the medical unit has good leadership, the POMR was instituted in this area. The decision was also based on the premise that change should begin where ego involvement is low, where success is assured, and where the nursing staff has the tools and the skills required, thus improving chances of success in other areas (reinforcement).

EVALUATION

> Evaluate
> effectiveness
> of
> action

An evaluation of the effectiveness of this planned change is determined by comparing the results with the previously established criteria (goals, behavioral objectives, and performance criteria). The problem-oriented system, launched in the medical intensive care unit, has spread to other units. Some of the units have developed their own defined data base, and each is progressing at its own pace. The specialty units are far ahead of the wards. This system was formally initiated with the arrival of new interns and residents, which made the transition easier.

Initially nurses charted as they always had, but separated their comments by problem number. After a few months of numbering entries according to the problem, the SOAP format was added. The system did not reach a totally acceptable level until all team members incorporated their entries into a single progress note.

Throughout the change process, the coordinator and inservice educator held classes for staff members, with practice in the POMR method of charting. Assistance was available on an individual basis and change relationships were established. The staff was given feedback at frequent intervals so that they could visualize their progress. Consultation with a nurse educator has been an ongoing process that has paid dividends. The institution was fortunate in having administrators and physicians committed to the POMR system.

When problem-oriented charting was first initiated, the nurses found that it required more time, thought, and effort on their part. Within weeks they became adept at analyzing complicated problems and at devising care and follow-up plans for each problem. Nurses acknowledged that they had improved their overall comprehension of the patients, and felt that their work became more meaningful and rewarding to them. There was also evidence of nurse acceptance. Requests were frequently made to incorporate this type of charting in other units.

Auditing records (a feedback loop) contributed to further improvement in recording data, which helped assure more thorough patient care management. These audits revealed the following: (1) nursing problems were being identified from a data base for each patient, (2) the content of the nursing care plans was a definite improvement from the traditional nursing care plan, (3) superfluous charting was reduced to a minimum, (4) the problem-oriented record facilitated documentation of skilled nursing care, (5) patient care had improved and POMR facilitated greater continuity of care, (6) significant patient data could be easily and accurately retrieved from charts, (7) the thinking processes of the nurse could be evaluated since each problem could be studied over a period of time, (8) problems could be examined individually or for their interrelationships, and (9) documentation of care was organized and logical.

Problem-oriented records eased the staffing problem since it became easier to substitute temporarily for another nurse. By reading the problem list and the progress notes the nurse could quickly grasp the nature of the patient's problems and the specific plan for each problem.

Revisions of the data base have undergone change, Kardexes have been revised, nursing care plans have been adapted to the problem list, and additional flow sheets have been added in some specialty units.

It is anticipated that it will take several years to change the entire hospital system. In addition, it has become clear that continual support at all levels is a requisite to maintaining staff interest, motivation, and satisfaction necessary for continued successful use of this concept.

From the data presented it appears that the decision of a health care team to incorporate the problem-oriented medical record as a quality control system has been essentially effective.

SUMMARY

The problem-oriented medical record (POMR) requires a multidisciplinary effort, frequent auditing to obtain feedback for correction and supplementation, effective leadership, and the collection of a standardized data base. The POMR system has implications for more comprehensive health care, for improved methods of educating health care practitioners, and for evaluating the quality of patient care.

Effective decision making through the use of the Claus-Bailey Systems Model for Problem Solution has been demonstrated by its application to the complex problem of selecting a quality control system. The nursing service director in an acute care center is responsible for assisting the staff in the decision making process. Leadership and decision making skill as well as skill in the use of problem-solving models can greatly enhance the director's managerial abilities through approaching problems in a systematic way before choosing and implementing a major change. Thus, the Claus-Bailey Systems Model for Problem Solution is recommended as an effective tool for directors of nursing service and staff members as they deal with complex patient care problems, seek solutions, and implement and evaluate the many changes needed to improve the quality of patient care.

REFERENCES

1. Alexander, E. L.: Nursing administration in the hospital health care system, St. Louis, 1972, The C. V. Mosby Co.
2. Armstrong, D. M., and Partridge, K. B.: Nursing excellence: A special challenge in complex settings, Nurs. Clin. North Am. **8:**209-218, 1973.
3. Bonkowsky, M. L.: Adapting the POMR to community child health care, Nurs. Outlook **20:**515-518, 1972.
4. Donabedian, A.: Some issues in evaluating the quality of nursing care, Am. J. Public Health, **59:**1833-1936, 1969.
5. Driggs, M. G.: Problem-directed and medical information systems, New York, 1973, Intercontinental Medical Book Corp.
6. Freeman, R. B.: Techniques of supervision in public health nursing, ed. 2, Philadelphia, 1949, W. B. Saunders Co.
7. Gold, H., Jackson, M., Sachs, B., and Van Meter, M. J.: Peer review—a working experiment, Nurs. Outlook **21:**634-636, 1973.
8. Lewin, K.: Field theory in social science, New York, 1951, Harper & Row, Publishers.
9. Mitchell, P. H.: A systematic nursing process record: the problem-oriented approach, Nurs. Forum **12:**187-210, 1973.
10. Myers, R. S.: Hospital statistics don't tell the truth, Mod. Hosp. **83:**53, 1954.
11. Peterson, G. C.: Do nursing administrators need advanced clinical preparation? Am. J. Nurs. **70:**297-303, 1970.
12. Phaneuf, M. C.: The nursing audit for evaluation of patient care, Nurs. Outlook **14:**51-54, 1966.
13. Phaneuf, M. C.: Analysis of a nursing audit, Nurs. Outlook **16:**57-60, 1968.
14. Phaneuf, M. C.: Quality of care: problems of measurement, Am. J. Public Health **59:**1827-1832, 1969.
15. Poland, M., English, N., Thornton, N., and Owens, D.: PETO: a system for assessing and meeting patient care needs, Am. J. Nurs. **70:**1479-1482, 1970.
16. Ramphal, M.: Peer review, Am. J. Nurs. **74:**63-67, 1974.
17. Rosenfeld, L. S.: Quality of medical care in hospitals, Am. J. Public Health **47:**856-865, 1957.
18. Stevens, B. J.: Analysis of trends in nursing care management, J. Nurs. Admin. **2:**12-17, 1972.
19. Weed, L. L.: Medical records, medical education, and patient care, Cleveland, Ohio, 1970, The Press of Case Western Reserve University.

SUGGESTED READINGS

Goldfinger, S. E.: The problem-oriented record: a critique from a believer, N. Engl. J. Med. **288:**606-608, 1973.
Graves, S.: Better records: first step to better quality, Mod. Hosp. **116:**105-108, 1971.
Hurst, J. W., and Walker, K. H.: The problem-

oriented system, New York, 1972, Medcom Press.

Phaneuf, M. C.: The nursing audit: profile for excellence, New York, 1972, Meridith Corp.

Schell, P. L., and Campbell, A. T.: POMR—not just another way to chart, Nurs. Outlook **20:**510-514, 1972.

Simmons, D. A.: Medical and hospital control systems, Boston, 1972, Little, Brown and Co.

Slee, V. N.: How to know if you have quality control, Hosp. Prog. **53:**38-43, 1972.

Thoma, D., and Pittman, K.: Evaluation of prob-lem-oriented nursing notes, J. Nurs. Admin. **2:**50-58, 1972.

Weed, L. L.: Medical records that guide and teach, N. Engl. J. Med. **278:**593-600, 652-657, 1968.

Weed, L. L.: Problem-oriented record as a basic tool in medical education, patient care and clinical research, Ann. Clin. Res. **3:**131-134, 1971.

Weed, L. L.: Quality control and the medical record, Arch. Inter. Med. **127:**101-105, 1971.

The diabetic should know everything that can be known about his ailment, its history, nature, how it develops, the problem it creates, and how it is treated. He should be able to distinguish medical fact from popular fancy, prejudice from sound practice. Knowing these things, he will be better able to cope with his disease every day of his life.

H. DOLGER AND B. SEEMAN*

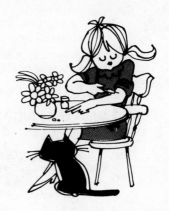

16 THE NURSE EDUCATOR IN A HEALTH MAINTENANCE ORGANIZATION

Developing and implementing an educational program for diabetic patients

CARELYN P. FYLLING, R.N., M.S.

The role of the diabetes nurse educator represents a new and emerging role for nurses in the delivery of health care. The diabetes nurse educator is prepared in an advanced nursing educational program granting graduate degrees. The preparation of the diabetes nurse educator is usually in the clinical specialty area of diabetes in the area of medical nursing, or in the chronic, long-term area with additional courses in teaching and curriculum design.

Diabetes is a chronic disease that afflicts an estimated four million people in the United States. In addition, there are over one million people who are unaware of having diabetes, and more than 5 percent of the population are destined to become diabetic. From a ranking of the seventh leading cause of death in 1964, diabetes is predicted to rank second by 1980, being outranked only by heart disease.

Since there is no known cure for diabetes, patients with this chronic disease need to be taught how to incorporate a health maintenance program of diet, medication and exercise into their daily lives. "Effective, efficient, preventive health care can only be carried out by an involved and informed patient."[3]

Health care delivery systems are beginning to recognize the need for a diabetes education program and are seeking information on how to establish a formalized program. Health maintenance organizations, which emphasize preventive health care, are among the first of the acute care centers to establish educational programs for diabetes patients.

This chapter describes how a diabetes nurse educator, charged with the task of de-

---

*From Dolger, H., and Seeman, B.: How to live with diabetes, New York, 1958; W. W. Horton Co.

signing a diabetes education program in a health maintenance organization, used the Claus-Bailey Model for Problem Solution to guide the problem solving and decision making processes inherent in the task. The model served as a step-by-step procedure and provided the nurse with a systematic, defensible way of developing a program to meet the needs of the patients, the health care system, and the community.

THE CASE OF DEVELOPING AN EDUCATIONAL PROGRAM FOR DIABETES PATIENTS AT URBAN MEDICAL CENTER

Urban Medical Center is composed of a 350-bed hospital and an adjacent twelve-story outpatient clinic building. The medical center is located in the western part of the United States in a community of 100,000 people. The patients served at the medical center usually enter the hospital under a prepaid insurance plan offered by the health maintenance organizations.

One floor of the clinic has been designated to house the Health Education Department. This floor is composed of offices, a classroom, a library, and audiovisual facilities. The offices of diabetes nurse educator and the dietitian, who is assisting in the program, are located on this floor. Funding for the program has been provided through the Urban Medical Center budget and from the patients' prepayment plan. Of the 110 physicians on the medical staff of the Center, 40 are internists and 15 are pediatricians whose diabetic patients are usually seen on an outpatient basis in the clinic.

A diabetes nurse educator with a master's degree who has had advanced preparation and considerable experience in the clinical area of diabetes has been employed to develop a diabetes education program for the medical center.

THE APPLICATION OF THE CLAUS-BAILEY MODEL FOR PROBLEM SOLUTION IN THE DEVELOPMENT OF A DIABETES EDUCATION PROGRAM

DEFINING THE OVERALL NEEDS, PURPOSES, AND GOALS

Define overall needs, purposes, goals

The overall needs, purposes, and goals of Urban Medical Center focus on providing patients with preventive, curative, and rehabilitative care using out-of-hospital care facilities as well as the in-hospital facilities.

The needs, purposes, and goals in the development of a diabetes education program. The overall *purpose* of a diabetes education program is to meet the *needs* of diabetic patients through instructional, support, and guidance services designed to enable patients with diabetes to function at a maximum level of wellness. Congruent with the overall goals of Urban Medical Center, the diabetes education program aims to assist diabetic patients to learn the medical facts about their disease; assist diabetic patients to adopt a therapeutic program of diet, medication, and exercise into their daily lives; prevent illness; and provide patients an opportunity to be active decision makers in their health care.

The discrepancy

Discrepancy

Although there is a need for diabetic patients to know how to apply knowledge about diet, medication, and exercise to daily living, there has not been an organized educational program at Urban Medical Center. The discrepancy thus appears to be between what is—a lack of an organized instructional diabetes program—and what should be—a need to develop a diabetes education program that will best meet the needs of the patient, the organization, and the community.

THE PROBLEM

<table>
<tr><td>
Define
problem
</td><td>

The basic problem is to develop a diabetes education program since there is no organized program within the hospital designed to educate diabetic patients about their disease. Individual teaching is done sporadically as the nurse caring for the patient finds time. The teaching includes only the bare essentials: urine testing, insulin administration, and occasionally foot care. Known diabetics in the community who are not hospital-
</td></tr>
</table>

ized have expressed feelings that they do not fully understand their diabetes or how to manage it. They would like to learn more. Because of a time factor, the physicians feel that they cannot do all the diabetes education themselves. The diabetes nurse educator is confronted with designing an institutional program to best meet the needs of diabetic patients.

CONSTRAINTS, CAPABILITIES, RESOURCES, AND CLAIMANT GROUPS

<table>
<tr><td>
Specify
constraints,
capabilities,
resources,
claimant
groups
</td><td>

The constraints and resources are presented in Fig. 16-1. The constraints are those forces that tend to resist or have negative effect on the development and implementation of a diabetes education program. The resources or capabilities use positive or pushing forces, which help the program become a reality. The two forces and their relative strength are illustrated in Fig. 16-1 as a modification of Lewin's force field analysis.[4]
</td></tr>
</table>

The major capabilities or resources are the educational facilities, the diabetes nurse educator, the dietitian, and the majority of the physicians. The primary constraint is the opposition of some of the physicians or claimant groups. Steps must be taken to strengthen the pushing forces and to weaken the constraints.

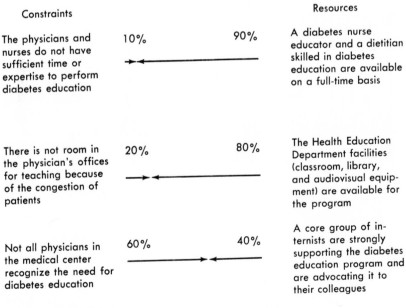

Constraints			Resources
The physicians and nurses do not have sufficient time or expertise to perform diabetes education	10%	90%	A diabetes nurse educator and a dietitian skilled in diabetes education are available on a full-time basis
There is not room in the physician's offices for teaching because of the congestion of patients	20%	80%	The Health Education Department facilities (classroom, library, and audiovisual equipment) are available for the program
Not all physicians in the medical center recognize the need for diabetes education	60%	40%	A core group of internists are strongly supporting the diabetes education program and are advocating it to their colleagues

Fig. 16-1. Analysis of constraints and resources.

THE APPROACH

> Specify approach to problem solution

A basic assumption in the health care of patients with diabetes is that diabetic patients, whether newly diagnosed or previously diagnosed, are candidates for diabetes education. Although diabetics may have received previous education, new products, procedures, theories, and research are continuously being developed, necessitating current knowledge for management. It is also assumed that education will help patients manage their disease better. For example, there will be fewer acute complications, fewer hospitalizations, and more effective treatment of chronic complications should they occur. In a study by Williams, "there was a positive correlation between knowledge and performance, i.e. the more patients know about the disease, the better they carry out recommended therapy."[6]

A patient-centered humanistic approach is the major focus in the development of the instructional program. This approach enables the diabetes nurse educator to individualize instruction as much as possible, to involve patients in the decision making process, and to endeavor to meet their needs. This approach can be based on McGregor's Theory Y.[5] Basically, McGregor assumes that people are naturally active, can set goals, enjoy striving, enjoy learning, enjoy creativity and innovation, have a respect for their fellow man, can improve their own methods of doing work, and are self-directed.

OBJECTIVES AND PERFORMANCE CRITERIA

> State behavioral objectives and performance criteria

The diabetes education program attempts to meet the instructional needs of diabetic patients by means of the following:

1. Providing educational services to diabetic patients and their families at a minimum cost through the prepayment plan
2. Providing the patients with convenient access to the education office
3. Providing the patients with the opportunity to schedule appointments with the diabetes nurse educator
4. Providing the patients with the opportunity to attend classes organized by the diabetes nurse educator
5. Providing patients with the opportunity for other medical center personnel to use the diabetes nurse educator as a consultant
6. Providing the patients with the opportunity to schedule appointments with the dietitian
7. Scheduling instruction at convenient times for patients

The diabetes education program was assessed on the following criteria:

1. The philosophy and objectives of the educational program have been developed and are available.
2. A job description for the diabetes nurse educator has been developed.
3. The roles of the diabetes nurse educator, dietitian, physicians, and patients in the program have been delineated.
4. The procedure for referring patients to the educational program and to their physicians has been determined.
5. An education schedule has been prepared and is available.
6. The referral procedure and education schedule have been made available to all physicians and nursing personnel in the Urban Medical Center.
7. Physicians are referring patients to the program.

8. Patients are attending the program.
9. The patients have demonstrated the success or lack of success of their education program verbally or through an assessment of their educational program.

ALTERNATIVE SOLUTIONS

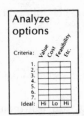

List alternative solutions
1. _____
2. _____
3. _____
4. _____
5. _____
6. _____
7. _____

In developing an educational program for diabetic patients the following alternatives should be considered:

1. Conduct a weekly full-day series of classes. These classes can be held in the Health Education Department classroom Monday through Friday from 7:30 AM to 4 PM. The series can be repeated each week. The diabetes nurse educator, dietitian, and selected physicians will each teach different topics on diabetes, hold individual and group conferences with the patients, and regulate the patients' medication, diet, and exercise during the week.

2. Schedule the referred patients for individual conferences and education sessions with the diabetes nurse educator and dietitian. The number of sessions a patient attends is determined by his management program, education needs, motivation, and ability to learn.

3. Conduct daytime classes each afternoon for 90 minutes. The diabetes nurse educator and dietitian will team teach the classes, covering a different topic each day. The 5-day series can be repeated each week. Inpatients and outpatients can attend the classes. While not in class, the diabetes nurse educator and dietitian should be available for individual appointments with patients and consultations with physicians and nursing personnel.

4. Conduct an evening class once a week for the first 4 weeks of the month; each evening class should last for 2½ hours. The diabetes nurse educator and dietitian team teach the classes, covering a different topic each week. The series can be repeated each month. Inpatients and outpatients can attend the classes. During the remainder of their working hours, the diabetes nurse educator and dietitian should be available for individual appointments with patients and consultations with physicians and nursing personnel.

5. Combine alternatives 3 and 4.

ANALYSIS OF OPTIONS

Analyze options
Criteria: Value Cost Feasibility Etc.
1.
2.
3.
4.
5.
6.
7.
Ideal: Hi Lo Hi

An analysis of the options is presented in Fig. 16-2. As noted in the analysis, the cost to the patient is "Lo" for each of the alternatives since the cost of the diabetes education program is included in the patients' prepaid health plan. The dietitian's availability for teaching is "Hi" in each of the alternatives presented.

In alternative 1, the classroom in the Health Education Department would not be available for the exclusive use of the diabetes education program since it is used for other patient and staff development classes. Consequently, it receives a low rating. The availability of the diabetes nurse educator also receives a low rating. She would be teaching classes all day and would not be available for individual patient appointments or consultations with health professionals. Patients would find it difficult to participate in full-day sessions, as work and school schedules usually take first priorities. A low rating for patient participation in classes is justified.

Alternative 2 indicates that five of the seven criteria are met. The unmet criteria indicate that the diabetes nurse educator would not be available for teaching classes or for

Ideal	Options					Criteria
	1	2	3	4	5	
Lo	(Lo)	(Lo)	(Lo)	(Lo)	(Lo)	Cost to patient
Hi	Lo	(Hi)	(Hi)	(Hi)	(Hi)	Education room availability
Hi	Lo	(Hi)	(Hi)	(Hi)	(Hi)	Diabetes nurse educator's availability for individual patient appointments
Hi	(Hi)	Lo	(Hi)	(Hi)	(Hi)	Diabetes nurse educator's availability for classes
Hi	Lo	Mod	(Hi)	(Hi)	(Hi)	Diabetes nurse educator's availability for consultations
Hi	(Hi)	(Hi)	(Hi)	(Hi)	(Hi)	Dietitian's availability
Hi	Lo	(Hi)	Lo	Lo	(Hi)	Time accessibility for patients
7	3	5	6	6	7	Score

Fig. 16-2. Analysis of the options.

consultation because her time would be devoted entirely to individual patient instruction.

In alternatives 3 and 4, all of the criteria are met with the exception of one, namely, the scheduled time for instructional classes for patients. Patients who work or attend school would probably not be able to attend daytime classes, and patients who are reluctant to travel at night would probably not attend the night classes.

Alternative 5 meets all the criterion measures, namely: (1) low cost, (2) availability of the classroom, (3) availability of the diabetes nurse educator to meet with patients on an individual basis, (4) availability of the diabetes nurse educator to conduct classes, (5) availability of the diabetes nurse educator to serve as consultant to nursing personnel and to consult with physicians, (6) availability of the dietitian, and (7) scheduling of classes at times when patients would find it convenient for them to attend.

DECISION RULES

Choose:
apply
decision
rules
A. _____
B. _____
C. _____
D. _____

The following decision rules will assist the diabetes nurse to develop an instructional program for diabetic patients.

1. The content of the diabetes education program will include the following: diet, tests of the urine, insulin and orally administered antidiabetic drugs, technique of insulin injection, care of the syringe and insulin, hypoglycemia, symptoms of uncontrolled diabetes, ketoacidosis, care of the feet (for older patients), and emergencies (recommendations by the American Diabetic Association).[1]

2. Diabetes education will be provided for the newly diagnosed diabetic patients in the hospital as well as those in the outpatient department.

3. The formalized instructional programs will be conducted when patients are available.

Table 3. Topics covered in the diabetes education schedule

Topic	Instructor	Topic	Instructor
Explanation of diabetes	Nurse	Labeling	Dietitian
Urine testing and recordkeeping	Nurse	Food for sick days	Dietitian
Diet introduction	Dietitian	Personal hygiene	Nurse
The exchange system of diet	Dietitian	Foot care	Nurse
Insulin injection procedure	Nurse	Exercise	Nurse
Equipment available	Nurse	Identification aides	Nurse
Care of equipment	Nurse	Community resources	Nurse
Insulin reactions and acidosis	Nurse	Dining in restaurants	Dietitian
Meal planning	Dietitian	Foods for special occasions	Dietitian

4. The diabetes education program will be conducted in such a way as to involve patients in decision making processes relative to their health maintenance program.

5. All diabetic patients seen by Urban Medical Center physicians will be eligible for the diabetes education program.

6. The diabetic patient's prepaid medical plan through the health maintenance organization will cover the cost of the diabetes education program.

IMPLEMENTATION

Control and implement decisions

Alternative 5 meets the criteria and conforms to the decision rules—conduct 90-minute daytime classes each afternoon, and conduct a weekly evening class for the first 4 weeks of the program.

To implement the decision, the following actions were taken: (1) the philosophy and objectives of the program were delineated, (2) the job description of the diabetes nurse educator was determined, (3) the roles of the dietitian, the patient, and the physician were determined, (4) the referral procedure was written and communicated, and (5) the education class schedule was prepared and approved.

The following education program was implemented: the education classes are held from 3 to 4:30 PM each afternoon, Monday through Friday and from 7 to 9:30 PM one evening a week for 4 weeks. The daytime series is repeated each week and the evening series each month. A different topic is taught by the diabetes nurse educator and dietician during each session. Topics covered in the education schedule are presented in Table 3.

Class sessions are held in the classroom within the Health Education Department. Both inpatients and outpatients, as well as family members, are invited to attend the classes. During the time the diabetes nurse educator is not teaching classes, she is available to see patients on an individual appointment basis, consult with the physicians regarding their diabetic patients, and consult with nursing personnel in the hospital and physicians' office building regarding diabetic patients.

Upon referral by the physician, the diabetes nurse educator interviews the diabetic patient, assesses his needs, establishes a teaching plan, teaches on a group or individual basis, evaluates the patient's progress, and revises the teaching plan as needed. Upon completion of the education program, a written evaluation relative to the patient's status is sent to his physician.

Brochures publicizing the diabetes education program and its services, the schedule of classes, and the procedures for attending classes have been distributed to all the physicians and nursing personnel in Urban Medical Center. One of the internists presented the format of the diabetes education program at a special meeting of the medical staff. The diabetes nurse educator and dietitian were invited to the meeting and introduced. The diabetes nurse educator presented the format of the educational program at a special meeting of the nursing staff and at its orientation program for new nursing staff members.

EVALUATION

Evaluate
effectiveness
of
action

The diabetes education program as it has been presented has met the previous stated criteria and a workable program has been established. Classes are being held in a location that is convenient for both outpatients and inpatients to reach. Classes are held at two separate times to accommodate patients who must work and thus can only attend evening classes, as well as patients who do not care to be away from home after dark and thus would rather attend during the daytime. There is no extra charge to the patient for these services. A quality program covering all areas of diabetes management is taught by skilled professionals. The patients receive individual as well as group attention from both the nurse and the dietitian. The diabetes nurse educator is also available for consultations with the physicians and nursing personnel of Urban Medical Center.*

SUMMARY

A formalized diabetes education program was developed and implemented in a health maintenance organization using the Claus-Bailey Systems Model as a tool. The diabetes nurse educator used the Model as guidelines and procedural steps in developing an educational program which would best meet the needs of patients, of the health care systems, and of the community. The Claus-Bailey Model proved invaluable in developing a program that is defensible and that appears to be highly effective.

---

*Since the program has only recently been implemented, total evaluation is not possible at this time.

REFERENCES

1. Allan, F.: Education of the diabetic patient, N. Engl. J. Med. **268:**93-95, 1963.
2. Dolger, H., and Seeman, B.: How to live with diabetes, New York, 1958, W. W. Horton Co.
3. Etzwiler, D.: Current status of patient education, J.A.M.A. **220:**583, 1972.
4. Lewin, K.: Field theory in social science, New York, 1951, Harper & Row, Publishers.
5. McGregor, K.: The human side of enterprise, New York, 1960, McGraw-Hill Book Co.
6. Williams, T., and others: The clinical picture of diabetic control, studies in four settings, Am. J. Public Health **57:**441-451, 1967.

SUGGESTED READINGS

Alston, K.: Hospital and community join in diabetic education program, Hospital Topics September:38-40, 1969.

Bowen, R., Rich, R., and Schlotfeldt, R.: Effects of organized instruction for patients with the diagnosis of diabetes mellitus, Nurs. Res. **10:** 151-159, 1961.

Cue, E.: The hospital pharmacist's role in health education, Am. J. Hosp. Pharm. **28:**697-700, 1971.

Etzwiler, D.: Who's teaching the diabetic? Diabetes **16:**111-117, 1967.

Etzwiler, D.: Education and management of the patient with diabetes mellitus, Elkhart, Ind., 1973, Ames Company, Division of Miles Laboratories, Inc.

Etzwiler, D., and others: Diabetes detection and education center: A regional resource for the practicing physician, Minn. Med. September: 1035-1039, 1970.

Hornback, M.: Diabetes mellitus—the nurse's role, Nurs. Clin. North Am. **5:**3-12, 1970.

Prater, B.: The diabetes center: A self-care living-in program, J. Am. Diet. Assoc. **64:**180-183, 1974.

Stern, S.: Educating the diabetic patient, J. La. State Med. Soc. **122:**332-336, 1970.

Ulrich, M., and Kelley, K.: Patient care includes teaching, Hospitals **46:**59-65, 1972.

Watkins, J., and others: A study of diabetic patients at home, Am. J. Public Health **57:**452-459, 1967.

Watkins, J., and Moss, F.: Confusion in the management of diabetes, Am. J. Nurs. **69:**521-524, 1969.

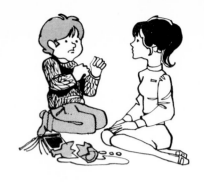

Nurses are disturbed because much of what they do is really not nursing. . . . They get the impression that administrators have forgotten that they are nurses, but view them as full-time managers and policemen.

M. MALONE*

17 THE PEDIATRIC CLINICAL SPECIALIST IN A COMMUNITY HOSPITAL

Reorganizing nursing care services

CAROLYN M. FONG, R.N., M.S.

Nurses as well as patients are becoming more vocal about the inadequacies of nursing care. New and expanded roles of nurses have enabled them to make an impact on the health care system in improving patient care services. Clinical specialists in particular are being effective change agents.

The emerging role of the clinical specialist is one of providing expert leadership in relation to nursing care, nursing education, and nursing research within a particular clinical specialty. The clinical specialist gives direct patient care, provides consultation, serves as a role model, and collaborates with nursing colleagues in establishing policies for the achievement of quality patient care.

In addition, there is a growing concern among clinical specialists to meet the needs of the nursing staff as well as the needs of patients. The specialist is beginning to be a facilitator in the promotion of a more stimulating work environment for nurses.

This chapter describes how a pediatric clinical specialist, charged with the task of dealing with the dissatisfaction of pediatric nurses, assisted them to define the problem and to make decisions. The Claus-Bailey model was utilized to analyze the problem and to select, implement, and evaluate a more effective method for organizing nursing care. The step-by-step procedure assisted the clinical specialist and the pediatric nurses in a community hospital to make rational, systematic judgments and to more effectively meet the needs of the child, the family, the nurse, and the community health care system.

THE CASE OF DISSATISFIED PEDIATRIC NURSES

Midland Community Hospital is a 250-bed hospital located in a community of 50,000 people. The people are from various ethnic, religious, and socioeconomic backgrounds represented by various professions, workers in industry, and ranchers.

---

*From Malone, M.: The dilemma of a professional in a bureaucracy, Nurs. Forum **3:**36-60, 1964.

The pediatric unit, Station 2E, is a 28-bed unit. The unit is divided into four medical teams: hematology and renal, cardiac, respiratory, and neurology. Each team consists of a resident, intern, and social worker. A dietitian, physicial therapist, inhalation therapist, and chaplain are available to all teams for consultation.

The family and the patient are an important component of this social system. Parents are invited to stay with the child during his hospitalization. The nurses view the child as a young, growing individual who needs stability and security in his environment. They feel that unfamiliar surroundings, procedures, routines, and the large number of health care workers are frightening to the child. Nurses also feel that a child needs a consistent nurturing person such as the parents and a specific nurse during hospitalization.

The nurses are predominantly young, white, middle-class females with recent baccalaureate degrees. The nursing component is separated into two teams under the head nurse. Within each team a modified type of functional nursing is practiced in which nurses are assigned various tasks. For example, aides collect urine specimens and take temperatures, LVNs take blood pressures, and RNs admit new patients and pass medications.

An element of team nursing is also practiced in that each team has a team leader who assigns patients and coordinates and supervises the day's activity of each team member. The patients are assigned to nurses according to geographical proximity and not according to the needs of the patients. Since the children are assigned to rooms according to age, sex, and disease entity, the team member may encounter a room with two groups of doctors making rounds, two lab technicians drawing blood, and four to six toddlers with their mothers. The teams of doctors, lab technicians, patients, and parents all have questions and needs which must be met.

Nursing services are fragmented. Patients receive nursing care from several different nurses during the day. The doctors complain because they do not know which nurse is taking care of their patients. One often hears: "Who is taking care of Johnny? What was his last temperature reading? Did he get his bone marrow done yet?" This entails the staff nurse's search for the nurse who is taking care of Johnny, the nurse who is taking temperatures, and for the team leader. Nurses appear more and more dissatisfied and frustrated. Furthermore, they are not using their nursing knowledge and skills to their fullest, and nursing care is centered on nursing tasks rather than on the child.

DEFINING THE OVERALL PURPOSES, NEEDS, AND GOALS

> Define overall needs, purposes, goals

The first step in dealing with the dissatisfaction of nurses defining the overall purposes, needs, and goals of nursing care.

Purpose. The overall purpose of pediatric nursing is to meet the physical, psychological, and social needs of each child. The responsibility for providing total, individualized, child-centered care is the central focus of each nurse.

Needs of the child. The first task in ego development is learning trust of the environment. Consistency, continuity, and sameness of experience are needed by the child to provide a rudimentary sense of ego identity.[2] Kutzman feels the child needs a consistent parent surrogate during hospitalization to supplement and ascertain that full attention is paid to the protective, nurturing, and comforting needs of the child.[4] The nurse must strive for an accepting, supporting, and continuous relationship with the mother; this includes the two sharing in the responsibility of child care. In summary, children and families need a consistent, warm, nurturing, and supporting nurse in order to deal with new situations, routines, and stresses while the child is hospitalized.

Needs of the nurse. Employees have inherent growth needs towards self-actualization that may be met by behavior which acknowledges achievement, gives recognition and responsibility, provides for advancement, and expands knowledge.[8] Factors closely related to the work itself, peer recognition or increased responsibility, contribute significantly to heighten satisfaction and increase motivation according to Herzburg.[3] Rewards for nurses come from seeing patients respond to their care. Nurses need a sense of task completion. Therefore continuity of care and comprehensiveness of care become important to nursing satisfaction.

Goals. The overall nursing goals for the pediatric nurses are:

1. To provide the children and their families with quality nursing care
2. To organize nursing care in such a way that the child is assured of continuous, comprehensive, and child-centered care
3. To assist the nursing service department to create a nursing enviornment to meet the professional and personal goals of the nurse

The discrepancy

Discrepancy

A discrepancy is the difference between "what is" and "what should be" happening in a particular situation. The nurses in pediatrics feel a painful discrepancy between "what is happening"—task-centered nursing—and "what should be happening"—child-centered nursing. Nurses want to be recognized as skilled professionals with the ability to deal with the patient's unique problem rather than to focus on procedures and tasks.

THE PROBLEM

Define problem

After determining the discrepancy, the basic problem is defined as the nurses' dissatisfaction with the method of organizing nursing care. The nurses want to be responsible for giving child-oriented direct care, thus practicing what they have learned. Instead they must perform task-oriented routine care dictated by the existing method of nursing care.

The nursing care method is centered on passing medications, reporting, assigning, and supervising other health workers. The nurses frequently feel that children need more individualized attention, so they will spend extra time to meet the specific needs of the patients. This necessitates nurses working overtime to do charting, ordering medications, and cleaning the medication room.

The pediatric nurses fell that a new mode of nursing care delivery is needed. They also feel that if their knowledge and expertise were more fully utilized, morale and job satisfaction among nurses would be higher. In addition, children and their families would receive more individualized, continuous, and comprehensive care.

THE APPROACH

Specify approach to problem solution

The approach to the problem is influenced by the clinical specialist's humanitarian set of values, which include the following: (1) people want to participate, be self-directive, and account for their own actions; (2) people want to grow, to develop, and to realize their full potential; and (3) people are self-controlled and self-motivated to do a good job. These values reflect the influence of McGregor's basic assumptions about man.[9]

The clinical specialists began by sharing personal observations and impressions during a nursing conference. She then posed the following questions: What did the pediatric nurses see as the problem? What are some possible solutions? The clinical specialist felt that once the nursing staff began sharing their feelings about their work problem they would be more committed to resolving it.

After a lengthy discussion, the nurses agreed to work together to find a new method

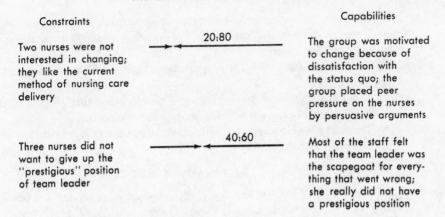

Fig. 17-1. Analysis of restraining and driving forces.

of delivering nursing care. A method needed to be found which would assure each nurse the freedom to function as a patient-centered professional.

CONSTRAINTS AND CAPABILITIES

Specify constraints, capabilities, resources, claimant groups

Bennis and Birnbaum propose that change takes place when an imbalance occurs between the sum of the restraining forces and the sum of the driving forces.[1] Such imbalance unfreezes the patterns: the level then changes until the opposing forces are again brought into equilibrium. An imbalance may occur through a change in the magnitude of a force, through a change in the direction of a force, or through the addition of a new force. The ratio of restraining to driving forces depicted in Fig. 17-1 were those perceived by the clinical specialists.

BEHAVIORAL OBJECTIVES

State behavioral objectives and performance criteria

The specific behavioral objective of the pediatric nurses was to develop a method of organizing patient care which would meet the needs of the child, the nurses, and the social system. A method for the delivery of nursing care needed to be found which would be child-centered, comprehensive, and continuous.

PERFORMANCE CRITERIA

The clinical specialist and the pediatric nurses decided on the performance criteria. The criteria generated were based on the needs and goals of the patient, the patient's family, the nurse, and the system. Observation and measurement of the performance criteria would assess the extent to which the nursing method was functioning. The criteria proposed included the following:

1. The nurse is responsible for the following patient-centered nursing activities: takes a nursing history; assesses patient's needs, symptoms, and problems; records and reports facts; initiates a nursing care plan for a 24-hour period; applies and executes nursing procedures and techniques; and evaluates the results of nursing intervention on patients assigned to her.

2. The nurse is accountable for independent nursing decisions carried out by the nursing process of assessing, planning, implementing, and evaluating the specific needs of the child and his family.

3. The nurse is assigned to the same patients each day for the duration of their hospitalization.

4. The nurse conducts patient-centered conferences with other staff members to coordinate a comprehensive interdisciplinary team approach.

5. The nurse is able to express satisfaction about the nursing care she provides.

6. The cost is less than $1,000.

ALTERNATIVE SOLUTIONS

List alternative solutions
1. _____
2. _____
3. _____
4. _____
5. _____
6. _____
7. _____

The nurses and the clinical specialist generated six possible ways of organizing nursing care: (1) functional nursing, (2) team nursing, (3) associate model, (4) case method, (5) primary nursing with head nurse, and (6) primary nursing with deletion of head nurse position.

The first alternative, functional nursing, was the existing method being used to organize nursing care.

In team nursing, nurses, LVNs, and aides would be put under the supervision and guidance of one nurse to provide nursing care to a large group of patients. Through the team nursing approach the unique abilities of each nurse could be utilized.

A third alternative was the traditional case method. However, the RN and nurse's aide have joint assignments as "associates," which is known as the associate model. The RN and aide share in the delivery of patient care, housekeeping, dietary, and transport functions for a caseload of patients according to their ability. The aide and the nurse bring to the patient care situation a different depth of understanding about human behavior and needs. The nurse may have a broader base of theoretical knowledge, the aide may have had more years of nursing experience.

The fourth alternative was to institute the case method, which is used in the nursing care of acutely ill patients. Each staff nurse is assigned a number of patients to whom she gives total care each day.

The fifth alternative was to consider primary nursing and to retain the position of the head nurse. Primary nursing is an organizational concept that facilitates coordinated individualized care for patients.[7] Nursing assignments enable primary nurses to be responsibile on a 24-hour basis for a caseload of patients during their hospitalization. The primary nurse makes decisions for the nursing care of patients and is accountable for them.

The sixth alternative was to institute primary nursing and delete the position of the head nurse. The head nurse becomes a primary nurse—she resumes giving direct child-oriented care. The coordination acitivities with families, the physician, and other departments are handled by each primary nurse.

ANALYSIS OF OPTIONS

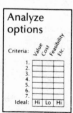

Analyze options

Criteria: Value / Cost / Feasibility / Etc.
1.
2.
3.
4.
5.
6.
7.
Ideal: Hi | Lo | Hi

An analysis of the options is presented in Fig. 17-2. The matrix compares the alternatives against specific criteria. The criteria were determined by the group from the needs, goals, and performance criteria previously stated. A score of high, moderate, or low is used to designate desirability for each criterion measure. Ideal scores have also been established.

The clinical specialist researched definitions for the criteria based

Ideal	Options						Criteria
	1	2	3	4	5	6	
Hi	Lo	Lo	(Hi)	(Hi)	(Hi)	(Hi)	Responsibility for patient-centered activities
Hi	Lo	Lo	Lo	(Hi)	(Hi)	(Hi)	Accountability for independent decisions
Hi	Lo	Lo	Mod	(Hi)	(Hi)	(Hi)	Continuity of care
Hi	(Hi)	(Hi)	(Hi)	Lo	(Hi)	(Hi)	Comprehensive interdisciplinary care
Hi	Lo	Lo	Lo	(Hi)	(Hi)	Lo	Using expertise of the nurse
Hi	Lo	Lo	Lo	Mod	(Hi)	Lo	Satisfaction of nurses
Lo	(Lo)	(Lo)	Hi	Hi	(Lo)	(Lo)	Cost
	2	2	2	4	7	5	Score

Fig. 17-2. Analysis of the options.

on current trends and policies. The criteria listed are in keeping with the growing trend of the nurse extending and defining her role in providing nursing care.

Responsibility for patient-centered nursing activities. Responsibility expresses the "oughts" or expectations of performance. One of the greatest challenges in nursing today is how to make it possible for nurses to carry full responsibility, over a continuous period of time, for the nursing care of patients. The associate, case, and primary methods offers nurses a high degree of responsibility for patient-centered nursing care. The nurse is assigned to a specific caseload of patients according to the needs of the child and the unique capabilities of the nurse. They are expected to deliver total, continuous, and individualized patient care.

Accountability for independent decisions. Accountability implies that the actual performance will be judged against expected performance. In a legalistic sense, accountability has a liability dimension that responsibility lacks. Demonstration of accountability is part of the nurse's basic value system in a helping profession. With group decision, as in the functional, team, and associate methods, the nurse is prevented from assuming individual accountability. Both primary models and the case model yield high accountability for independent nursing decisions. The assessment, diagnosis, and solution of nursing problems are not divided among various members.

Continuity of care. Communication between the nurse and patient must be kept as uninterrupted as possible to have continuous patient-centered care. More continuous service occurs when one person is involved in the care of a particular patient. The case model and primary model, in which one nurse is responsible for coordinating patient care for a specified time, has the highest probability of continuous one-to-one nurse-patient interaction.

Comprehensive interdisciplinary care. Comprehensiveness of health care means caring for all aspects of the individual on the health-illness continuum. It is necessary to tap the knowledge of various health disciplines to meet the physical, psychological, social, and spiritual needs of the patient. The functional, team, and associate models offer high comprehensive care since more individuals with specialized skills are involved with the child. Patient-centered conferences are necessary for collaborating and assessing each child's individual needs. With the primary nurse at the bedside fully accountable for nursing care for 24 hours, there is more effective communication between the nurse and other health disciplines. This assures the child of more comprehensive and coordinated care.

Using the expertise of the nurse. Functional and team nursing are task-oriented, fragment patient care, and do not use the knowledge and skills of the nurse. Nurses are managers, kept away from patient care. The primary model with the deletion of a head nurse does not use the expertise of the head nurse. The staff nurses wanted a strong leader available as a consultant, resource person, coordinator, and validator to meet the needs of both patients and nurses. The case method and the primary nursing model with the head nurse were highly feasible because they foster the utilization of the nurse's knowledge and skills and focus on greater nursing autonomy and development.

Satisfaction of nurses. When nurses are encouraged to practice patient-oriented nursing and to increase their nursing decision making skills by using them to assist patients, their major dissatisfaction with the organization of nursing care will be overcome. Nurses want to be recognized as skilled professionals with the ability to deal with the patient's unique problems. In the primary method with the head nurse there is a high degree of satisfaction with the nursing care provided because the environment meets the needs of the nurse for professional recognition, responsibility, and development. Primary nursing with the deletion of the head nurse is not satisfactory to the nurses because they no longer have an effective leader available to influence and facilitate their professional growth and development.

Cost. In the case and associate models, the need for additional nurses and nurse's aides increases the cost above $1,000. The functional, team, and primary models offer no increase in cost to the organization. The functional and team methods delegate work so that each worker's skill can be efficiently utilized. According to Manthey, in primary nursing additional RNs are not needed.[6] The same amount of care is planned and given in primary nursing as in team nursing.

As shown in Fig. 17-2, the two primary nursing models are only two points apart. At this point, decision rules must be generated and applied.

DECISION RULES

Choose:
apply
decision
rules
A. _____
B. _____
C. _____
D. _____

Four major decision rules were generated as guidelines in the decision sequence.

1. The nurses on the pediatric unit in consultation with the clinical specialist must clearly define the problem and resolve it.

2. The unit nurses and the clinical specialist must use a systematic approach in the decision making process for problem solution.

3. The alternative must be financially feasible.

4. The method of organizing nursing care that meets the largest number of criteria must also be agreed upon by the majority of nurses on the unit.

The nurses, when confronted with the decision situation, selected the best option according to the decision rules. The first and second decision rules will be met by using the Claus-Bailey Model for Problem Solution. The application of the third rule showed Options 5 and 6 to be financially feasible to the entire social system.

Looking at Fig. 17-2 and comparing Options 5 and 6 to the fourth rule, Option 5 meets the largest number of criteria. Although both options offer high accountability and responsibility, high continuity, and high comprehensive interdisciplinary patient services, the expertise of the head nurse is not utilized in Option 6. The nurses respect and trust the role of the head nurse. They value the opportunity to validate their needs and the patient's needs with a strong leader. Under the leadership of the head nurse is a cohesive peer group that can identify and solve staff and patient problems. Option 5, maintaining the role of the head nurse, is much more satisfactory to the nurses than Option 6.

The best alternative is primary nursing because it is most acceptable to the nurses, patients, and administrators. Primary nursing offers the concept of total accountability for nursing care vested in one nurse. It presents the best comprehensiveness and continuity of care to meet the individual needs of the child within the resources of the system. It also offers a framework for development of professional practice for the nurse.

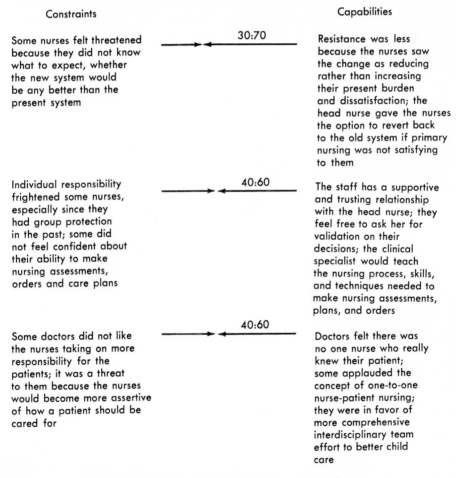

Constraints		Capabilities
Some nurses felt threatened because they did not know what to expect, whether the new system would be any better than the present system	30:70	Resistance was less because the nurses saw the change as reducing rather than increasing their present burden and dissatisfaction; the head nurse gave the nurses the option to revert back to the old system if primary nursing was not satisfying to them
Individual responsibility frightened some nurses, especially since they had group protection in the past; some did not feel confident about their ability to make nursing assessments, orders and care plans	40:60	The staff has a supportive and trusting relationship with the head nurse; they feel free to ask her for validation on their decisions; the clinical specialist would teach the nursing process, skills, and techniques needed to make nursing assessments, plans, and orders
Some doctors did not like the nurses taking on more responsibility for the patients; it was a threat to them because the nurses would become more assertive of how a patient should be cared for	40:60	Doctors felt there was no one nurse who really knew their patient; some applauded the concept of one-to-one nurse-patient nursing; they were in favor of more comprehensive interdisciplinary team effort to better child care

Fig. 17-3. Analysis of restraining and driving forces.

CONSTRAINTS AND CAPABILITIES

Specify constraints, capabilities, resources, claimant groups

Before the group came to a final decision to implement primary nursing they retraced steps and again looked at constraints and capabilities. These are presented in Fig. 17-3. It is important to reduce the resistance to change if primary nursing is to be accomplished with minimal stress.

IMPLEMENTATION

Control and implement decisions

To implement primary nursing the nurses needed support from administration and other disciplines. Adequate communication and understanding were critical for acceptance. The clinical specialist photocopied the existing articles on primary care nursing and distributed them to nurses, doctors, and other health professionals. The clinical specialist also met with different groups to explain and discuss the goals of the staff and reasons for the change. Patient-centered conferences with interdisciplinary members participating were initiated.

A nine-member task force committee from the three nursing shifts was organized by the clinical specialist, who served as consultant. The task force prepared the specific objectives of primary nursing in their system and the specific behavioral objectives of the primary nurse.

The clinical specialist recommended that each primary nurse be responsible for the total nursing care of an assigned group of three to five patients. She would take nursing histories; assess, plan, implement, and evaluate care plans; attend ward rounds with physicians and nurses; do patient and family education; take vital signs; do discharge planning; administer medications; and perform treatments for specific patients. Extended functions such as home visits, physical examinations, and other services would be initiated according to the skills and ability of the nurse. These extended functions would stimulate primary nurses to learn and continually improve their holistic approach to patient care.

The clinical specialist would initially also have a patient load to act as a role model and resource to the nurses. She would begin classes on the nursing process, interviewing, physical assessment, and other subjects as needed.

The head nurse's functions would consist of responsibility for the 24-hour functioning and management of the unit, assignment of patients to personnel on the basis of assessed needs of the child and family, as well as the interest and unique capabilities of the nurses, collaboration with the clinical specialist to enhance staff development while serving as a resource person, and stimulation of intellectual activities in the staff and positive reinforcement for child-centered care.

The nurse's relationship with patients would remain "primary" even when she rotates to an afternoon or night duty. When the primary nurse would be off duty, the nurse caring for her patients would follow the nursing care plan which the primary nurse had developed. The nursing care plan would outline the nursing actions to be taken on a 24-hour basis for the duration of the hospitalization. The primary nurse would be responsible for any fundamental change in the design of the plan, although other nurses may change parts of the care plan to reflect changes in the patient's needs.

In primary nursing, each nurse is accountable for decisions made concerning patient care. Periodic care review conferences would be planned as a mechanism for nurses to validate their decisions with their colleagues and maintain quality control.

RESULTS

Results

The primary care system has been in effect on the unit for 1 month at the time this is written. During this period, several positive changes have occurred. First, each nurse had taken more responsibility and accountability for her patients. Nurses are making nursing decisions and accepting responsibility for these decisions. There is increased interest in continuity and comprehensiveness of patient-centered care. The children are being followed by the same nurses throughout their stay. There is a more trust and in-depth relationship between the nurse and the child. Direct communication between families and staff members has increased.

The interdisciplinary teams work together to attain comprehensive care for the patient. For instance, the night shift nurses often stay after hours to contribute their observations to the entire team during ward rounds. The primary nurse communicates directly with the physician or other members of the health team, and the other members communicate directly with her about the patient's needs. This fosters a colleague relationship, and a more vital interest in what is happening to the child.

The head nurse has fostered a work environment which encourages innovative nursing practice and professional growth and development. It is an atmosphere in which the nurses feel free to learn, to take risks, to grow, and to use their knowledge and skills.

EVALUATION

Evaluate
and
implement
decisions

Since primary nursing has only recently been implemented, its effectiveness has not been evaluated. The clinical specialist has assumed responsibility for educating the nursing staff about primary nursing, implementing the process, and evaluating the rate of progress and effectiveness after implementation. A systematic evaluation program is in the process of development.

SUMMARY

The clinical specialist in a community hospital is frequently called upon to assist the director of nursing service in the management of complex problems related to patient care. The Claus-Bailey Model has proved invaluable as a systematic way of defining problems, seeking solutions, predicting consequences of various alternatives, implementing change, and evaluating results.

In the case presented, primary nursing proved to the the most effective method for organizing nursing care to assure continuous, comprehensive, individualized, child-centered care. Assuming that nurses work in hospitals because of a basic motivation to help people, provisions must be made to provide nurses with satisfactions from their professional endeavors. Nurses need the satisfaction which comes from giving individualized patient care, and want to give patients the continuous and comprehensive care they deserve.

REFERENCES

1. Bennis, W., Benne, K., and Chin, R.: Planning of change, New York, 1969, Holt, Rinehart & Winston.
2. Erickson, E.: Childhood and society, ed. 2, New York, 1963, Norton & Co.
3. Herzburg, F.: Work and the nature of man, Cleveland, 1966, World Publishing Co.
4. Kutzman, L.: Some factors influencing a young child's mastery of hospitalization, Nurs. Clin. N. Amer. **7:**13-26, 1972.
5. Malone, M.: The dilemma of a professional in a bureaucracy, Nurs. Forum **3:**36-40, 1964.
6. Manthey, M., Ciske, K., Robertson, P., and Harris, I.: Primary nursing, Nurs. Forum **9:**65-89, 1970.
7. Marram, G., Schlegel, M., and Bevis, E.: Primary nursing, St. Louis, 1974, The C. V. Mosby Co.
8. Maslow, A.: Maturation and personality, New York, 1954, Harper & Row, Publishers.
9. McGregor, D.: The human side of enterprise, New York 1960, McGraw-Hill Book Co.

SUGGESTED READINGS

Bakke, K.: Primary nursing: Perceptions of a staff nurse, Am. J. Nurs. **73:**1432-1435, 1973.
Ciske, K.: Primary nursing: Evaluation, Am. J. Nurs. **73:**1437-1439, 1973.
Logsdon, A.: Why primary nursing? Nurs. Clin. N. Amer. **8:**283-291, 1973.
Manthey, M.: Primary care is alive and well in the hospital, Am. J. Nurs. **73:**83-87, 1973.
Manthey, M., Ciske, K., Robertson, P., and Harris, I.: Primary nursing: A return to the concept of "my nurse" and "my patient," Nurs. Forum **9:**65-83, 1970.
Manthey, M., and Kramer, M.: A dialogue on primary nursing between Marie Manthey and Marlene Kramer, Nurs. Forum **9:**356-379, 1971.
Marram, G.: Innovation on Four Tower West: What happened? Am. J. Nurs. **73:**814-816, 1973.
Page, M.: Primary nursing: Perceptions of a head nurse, Am. J. Nurs. **73:**1435-1437, 1973.
Schlegel, M.: Innovation on Four Tower West: How? Am. J. Nurs. **73:**811-813, 1973.
Schutt, B.: Spot check on primary care nursing, Am. J. Nurs. **72:**1996-2003, 1972.

INDEX